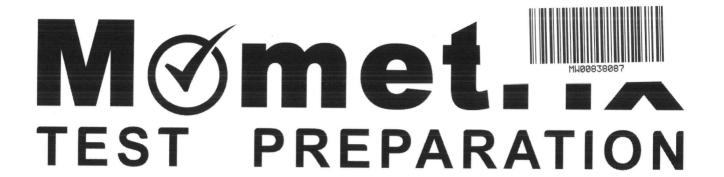

NPTAE

Secrets Study Guide
Part 1 of 2

DEAR FUTURE EXAM SUCCESS STORY

First of all, **THANK YOU** for purchasing Mometrix study materials!

Second, congratulations! You are one of the few determined test-takers who are committed to doing whatever it takes to excel on your exam. **You have come to the right place.** We developed these study materials with one goal in mind: to deliver you the information you need in a format that's concise and easy to use.

In addition to optimizing your guide for the content of the test, we've outlined our recommended steps for breaking down the preparation process into small, attainable goals so you can make sure you stay on track.

We've also analyzed the entire test-taking process, identifying the most common pitfalls and showing how you can overcome them and be ready for any curveball the test throws you.

Standardized testing is one of the biggest obstacles on your road to success, which only increases the importance of doing well in the high-pressure, high-stakes environment of test day. Your results on this test could have a significant impact on your future, and this guide provides the information and practical advice to help you achieve your full potential on test day.

Your success is our success

We would love to hear from you! If you would like to share the story of your exam success or if you have any questions or comments in regard to our products, please contact us at **800-673-8175** or **support@mometrix.com**.

Thanks again for your business and we wish you continued success!

Sincerely,
The Mometrix Test Preparation Team

> **Need more help? Check out our flashcards at:**
> **http://MometrixFlashcards.com/NPTE**

TABLE OF CONTENTS

0-27

31-40

27-35

Introduction

Thank you for purchasing this resource! You have made the choice to prepare yourself for a test that could have a huge impact on your future, and this guide is designed to help you be fully ready for test day. Obviously, it's important to have a solid understanding of the test material, but you also need to be prepared for the unique environment and stressors of the test, so that you can perform to the best of your abilities.

For this purpose, the first section that appears in this guide is the **Secret Keys**. We've devoted countless hours to meticulously researching what works and what doesn't, and we've boiled down our findings to the five most impactful steps you can take to improve your performance on the test. We start at the beginning with study planning and move through the preparation process, all the way to the testing strategies that will help you get the most out of what you know when you're finally sitting in front of the test.

We recommend that you start preparing for your test as far in advance as possible. However, if you've bought this guide as a last-minute study resource and only have a few days before your test, we recommend that you skip over the first two Secret Keys since they address a long-term study plan.

If you struggle with **test anxiety**, we strongly encourage you to check out our recommendations for how you can overcome it. Test anxiety is a formidable foe, but it can be beaten, and we want to make sure you have the tools you need to defeat it.

Secret Key #1 – Plan Big, Study Small

There's a lot riding on your performance. If you want to ace this test, you're going to need to keep your skills sharp and the material fresh in your mind. You need a plan that lets you review everything you need to know while still fitting in your schedule. We'll break this strategy down into three categories.

Information Organization

Start with the information you already have: the official test outline. From this, you can make a complete list of all the concepts you need to cover before the test. Organize these concepts into groups that can be studied together, and create a list of any related vocabulary you need to learn so you can brush up on any difficult terms. You'll want to keep this vocabulary list handy once you actually start studying since you may need to add to it along the way.

Time Management

Once you have your set of study concepts, decide how to spread them out over the time you have left before the test. Break your study plan into small, clear goals so you have a manageable task for each day and know exactly what you're doing. Then just focus on one small step at a time. When you manage your time this way, you don't need to spend hours at a time studying. Studying a small block of content for a short period each day helps you retain information better and avoid stressing over how much you have left to do. You can relax knowing that you have a plan to cover everything in time. In order for this strategy to be effective though, you have to start studying early and stick to your schedule. Avoid the exhaustion and futility that comes from last-minute cramming!

Study Environment

The environment you study in has a big impact on your learning. Studying in a coffee shop, while probably more enjoyable, is not likely to be as fruitful as studying in a quiet room. It's important to keep distractions to a minimum. You're only planning to study for a short block of time, so make the most of it. Don't pause to check your phone or get up to find a snack. It's also important to **avoid multitasking**. Research has consistently shown that multitasking will make your studying dramatically less effective. Your study area should also be comfortable and well-lit so you don't have the distraction of straining your eyes or sitting on an uncomfortable chair.

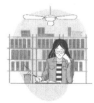 The time of day you study is also important. You want to be rested and alert. Don't wait until just before bedtime. Study when you'll be most likely to comprehend and remember. Even better, if you know what time of day your test will be, set that time aside for study. That way your brain will be used to working on that subject at that specific time and you'll have a better chance of recalling information.

Finally, it can be helpful to team up with others who are studying for the same test. Your actual studying should be done in as isolated an environment as possible, but the work of organizing the information and setting up the study plan can be divided up. In between study sessions, you can discuss with your teammates the concepts that you're all studying and quiz each other on the details. Just be sure that your teammates are as serious about the test as you are. If you find that your study time is being replaced with social time, you might need to find a new team.

2

Secret Key #2 – Make Your Studying Count

You're devoting a lot of time and effort to preparing for this test, so you want to be absolutely certain it will pay off. This means doing more than just reading the content and hoping you can remember it on test day. It's important to make every minute of study count. There are two main areas you can focus on to make your studying count.

Retention

It doesn't matter how much time you study if you can't remember the material. You need to make sure you are retaining the concepts. To check your retention of the information you're learning, try recalling it at later times with minimal prompting. Try carrying around flashcards and glance at one or two from time to time or ask a friend who's also studying for the test to quiz you.

To enhance your retention, look for ways to put the information into practice so that you can apply it rather than simply recalling it. If you're using the information in practical ways, it will be much easier to remember. Similarly, it helps to solidify a concept in your mind if you're not only reading it to yourself but also explaining it to someone else. Ask a friend to let you teach them about a concept you're a little shaky on (or speak aloud to an imaginary audience if necessary). As you try to summarize, define, give examples, and answer your friend's questions, you'll understand the concepts better and they will stay with you longer. Finally, step back for a big picture view and ask yourself how each piece of information fits with the whole subject. When you link the different concepts together and see them working together as a whole, it's easier to remember the individual components.

Finally, practice showing your work on any multi-step problems, even if you're just studying. Writing out each step you take to solve a problem will help solidify the process in your mind, and you'll be more likely to remember it during the test.

Modality

Modality simply refers to the means or method by which you study. Choosing a study modality that fits your own individual learning style is crucial. No two people learn best in exactly the same way, so it's important to know your strengths and use them to your advantage.

For example, if you learn best by visualization, focus on visualizing a concept in your mind and draw an image or a diagram. Try color-coding your notes, illustrating them, or creating symbols that will trigger your mind to recall a learned concept. If you learn best by hearing or discussing information, find a study partner who learns the same way or read aloud to yourself. Think about how to put the information in your own words. Imagine that you are giving a lecture on the topic and record yourself so you can listen to it later.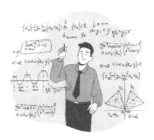

For any learning style, flashcards can be helpful. Organize the information so you can take advantage of spare moments to review. Underline key words or phrases. Use different colors for different categories. Mnemonic devices (such as creating a short list in which every item starts with the same letter) can also help with retention. Find what works best for you and use it to store the information in your mind most effectively and easily.

3

Secret Key #3 – Practice the Right Way

Your success on test day depends not only on how many hours you put into preparing, but also on whether you prepared the right way. It's good to check along the way to see if your studying is paying off. One of the most effective ways to do this is by taking practice tests to evaluate your progress. Practice tests are useful because they show exactly where you need to improve. Every time you take a practice test, pay special attention to these three groups of questions:

- The questions you got wrong
- The questions you had to guess on, even if you guessed right
- The questions you found difficult or slow to work through

This will show you exactly what your weak areas are, and where you need to devote more study time. Ask yourself why each of these questions gave you trouble. Was it because you didn't understand the material? Was it because you didn't remember the vocabulary? Do you need more repetitions on this type of question to build speed and confidence? Dig into those questions and figure out how you can strengthen your weak areas as you go back to review the material.

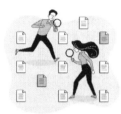 Additionally, many practice tests have a section explaining the answer choices. It can be tempting to read the explanation and think that you now have a good understanding of the concept. However, an explanation likely only covers part of the question's broader context. Even if the explanation makes perfect sense, **go back and investigate** every concept related to the question until you're positive you have a thorough understanding.

As you go along, keep in mind that the practice test is just that: practice. Memorizing these questions and answers will not be very helpful on the actual test because it is unlikely to have any of the same exact questions. If you only know the right answers to the sample questions, you won't be prepared for the real thing. **Study the concepts** until you understand them fully, and then you'll be able to answer any question that shows up on the test.

It's important to wait on the practice tests until you're ready. If you take a test on your first day of study, you may be overwhelmed by the amount of material covered and how much you need to learn. Work up to it gradually.

On test day, you'll need to be prepared for answering questions, managing your time, and using the test-taking strategies you've learned. It's a lot to balance, like a mental marathon that will have a big impact on your future. Like training for a marathon, you'll need to start slowly and work your way up. When test day arrives, you'll be ready.

Start with the strategies you've read in the first two Secret Keys—plan your course and study in the way that works best for you. If you have time, consider using multiple study resources to get different approaches to the same concepts. It can be helpful to see difficult concepts from more than one angle. Then find a good source for practice tests. Many times, the test website will suggest potential study resources or provide sample tests.

4

Practice Test Strategy

If you're able to find at least three practice tests, we recommend this strategy:

UNTIMED AND OPEN-BOOK PRACTICE

Take the first test with no time constraints and with your notes and study guide handy. Take your time and focus on applying the strategies you've learned.

TIMED AND OPEN-BOOK PRACTICE

Take the second practice test open-book as well, but set a timer and practice pacing yourself to finish in time.

TIMED AND CLOSED-BOOK PRACTICE

Take any other practice tests as if it were test day. Set a timer and put away your study materials. Sit at a table or desk in a quiet room, imagine yourself at the testing center, and answer questions as quickly and accurately as possible.

Keep repeating timed and closed-book tests on a regular basis until you run out of practice tests or it's time for the actual test. Your mind will be ready for the schedule and stress of test day, and you'll be able to focus on recalling the material you've learned.

Secret Key #4 – Pace Yourself

Once you're fully prepared for the material on the test, your biggest challenge on test day will be managing your time. Just knowing that the clock is ticking can make you panic even if you have plenty of time left. Work on pacing yourself so you can build confidence against the time constraints of the exam. Pacing is a difficult skill to master, especially in a high-pressure environment, so **practice is vital**.

Set time expectations for your pace based on how much time is available. For example, if a section has 60 questions and the time limit is 30 minutes, you know you have to average 30 seconds or less per question in order to answer them all. Although 30 seconds is the hard limit, set 25 seconds per question as your goal, so you reserve extra time to spend on harder questions. When you budget extra time for the harder questions, you no longer have any reason to stress when those questions take longer to answer.

Don't let this time expectation distract you from working through the test at a calm, steady pace, but keep it in mind so you don't spend too much time on any one question. Recognize that taking extra time on one question you don't understand may keep you from answering two that you do understand later in the test. If your time limit for a question is up and you're still not sure of the answer, mark it and move on, and come back to it later if the time and the test format allow. If the testing format doesn't allow you to return to earlier questions, just make an educated guess; then put it out of your mind and move on.

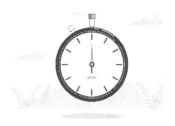

On the easier questions, be careful not to rush. It may seem wise to hurry through them so you have more time for the challenging ones, but it's not worth missing one if you know the concept and just didn't take the time to read the question fully. Work efficiently but make sure you understand the question and have looked at all of the answer choices, since more than one may seem right at first.

Even if you're paying attention to the time, you may find yourself a little behind at some point. You should speed up to get back on track, but do so wisely. Don't panic; just take a few seconds less on each question until you're caught up. Don't guess without thinking, but do look through the answer choices and eliminate any you know are wrong. If you can get down to two choices, it is often worthwhile to guess from those. Once you've chosen an answer, move on and don't dwell on any that you skipped or had to hurry through. If a question was taking too long, chances are it was one of the harder ones, so you weren't as likely to get it right anyway.

On the other hand, if you find yourself getting ahead of schedule, it may be beneficial to slow down a little. The more quickly you work, the more likely you are to make a careless mistake that will affect your score. You've budgeted time for each question, so don't be afraid to spend that time. Practice an efficient but careful pace to get the most out of the time you have.

6

Secret Key #5 – Have a Plan for Guessing

When you're taking the test, you may find yourself stuck on a question. Some of the answer choices seem better than others, but you don't see the one answer choice that is obviously correct. What do you do?

The scenario described above is very common, yet most test takers have not effectively prepared for it. Developing and practicing a plan for guessing may be one of the single most effective uses of your time as you get ready for the exam.

In developing your plan for guessing, there are three questions to address:

- When should you start the guessing process?
- How should you narrow down the choices?
- Which answer should you choose?

When to Start the Guessing Process

Unless your plan for guessing is to select C every time (which, despite its merits, is not what we recommend), you need to leave yourself enough time to apply your answer elimination strategies. Since you have a limited amount of time for each question, that means that if you're going to give yourself the best shot at guessing correctly, you have to decide quickly whether or not you will guess.

Of course, the best-case scenario is that you don't have to guess at all, so first, see if you can answer the question based on your knowledge of the subject and basic reasoning skills. Focus on the key words in the question and try to jog your memory of related topics. Give yourself a chance to bring the knowledge to mind, but once you realize that you don't have (or you can't access) the knowledge you need to answer the question, it's time to start the guessing process.

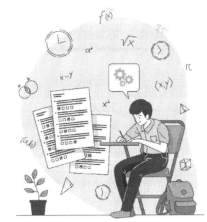

It's almost always better to start the guessing process too early than too late. It only takes a few seconds to remember something and answer the question from knowledge. Carefully eliminating wrong answer choices takes longer. Plus, going through the process of eliminating answer choices can actually help jog your memory.

Summary: Start the guessing process as soon as you decide that you can't answer the question based on your knowledge.

7

How to Narrow Down the Choices

The next chapter in this book (**Test-Taking Strategies**) includes a wide range of strategies for how to approach questions and how to look for answer choices to eliminate. You will definitely want to read those carefully, practice them, and figure out which ones work best for you. Here though, we're going to address a mindset rather than a particular strategy.

Your odds of guessing an answer correctly depend on how many options you are choosing from.

Number of options left	5	4	3	2	1
Odds of guessing correctly	20%	25%	33%	50%	100%

You can see from this chart just how valuable it is to be able to eliminate incorrect answers and make an educated guess, but there are two things that many test takers do that cause them to miss out on the benefits of guessing:

- Accidentally eliminating the correct answer
- Selecting an answer based on an impression

We'll look at the first one here, and the second one in the next section.

To avoid accidentally eliminating the correct answer, we recommend a thought exercise called **the $5 challenge**. In this challenge, you only eliminate an answer choice from contention if you are willing to bet $5 on it being wrong. Why $5? Five dollars is a small but not insignificant amount of money. It's an amount you could afford to lose but wouldn't want to throw away. And while losing

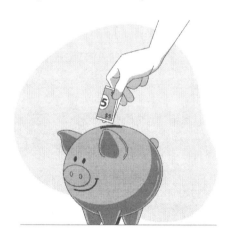

$5 once might not hurt too much, doing it twenty times will set you back $100. In the same way, each small decision you make—eliminating a choice here, guessing on a question there—won't by itself impact your score very much, but when you put them all together, they can make a big difference. By holding each answer choice elimination decision to a higher standard, you can reduce the risk of accidentally eliminating the correct answer.

The $5 challenge can also be applied in a positive sense: If you are willing to bet $5 that an answer choice *is* correct, go ahead and mark it as correct.

Summary: Only eliminate an answer choice if you are willing to bet $5 that it is wrong.

Which Answer to Choose

You're taking the test. You've run into a hard question and decided you'll have to guess. You've eliminated all the answer choices you're willing to bet $5 on. Now you have to pick an answer. Why do we even need to talk about this? Why can't you just pick whichever one you feel like when the time comes?

The answer to these questions is that if you don't come into the test with a plan, you'll rely on your impression to select an answer choice, and if you do that, you risk falling into a trap. The test writers know that everyone who takes their test will be guessing on some of the questions, so they intentionally write wrong answer choices to seem plausible. You still have to pick an answer though, and if the wrong answer choices are designed to look right, how can you ever be sure that you're not falling for their trap? The best solution we've found to this dilemma is to take the decision out of your hands entirely. Here is the process we recommend:

Once you've eliminated any choices that you are confident (willing to bet $5) are wrong, select the first remaining choice as your answer.

Whether you choose to select the first remaining choice, the second, or the last, the important thing is that you use some preselected standard. Using this approach guarantees that you will not be enticed into selecting an answer choice that looks right, because you are not basing your decision on how the answer choices look.

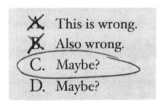

This is not meant to make you question your knowledge. Instead, it is to help you recognize the difference between your knowledge and your impressions. There's a huge difference between thinking an answer is right because of what you know, and thinking an answer is right because it looks or sounds like it should be right.

Summary: To ensure that your selection is appropriately random, make a predetermined selection from among all answer choices you have not eliminated.

Test-Taking Strategies

This section contains a list of test-taking strategies that you may find helpful as you work through the test. By taking what you know and applying logical thought, you can maximize your chances of answering any question correctly!

It is very important to realize that every question is different and every person is different: no single strategy will work on every question, and no single strategy will work for every person. That's why we've included all of them here, so you can try them out and determine which ones work best for different types of questions and which ones work best for you.

Question Strategies

⊘ READ CAREFULLY

Read the question and the answer choices carefully. Don't miss the question because you misread the terms. You have plenty of time to read each question thoroughly and make sure you understand what is being asked. Yet a happy medium must be attained, so don't waste too much time. You must read carefully and efficiently.

⊘ CONTEXTUAL CLUES

Look for contextual clues. If the question includes a word you are not familiar with, look at the immediate context for some indication of what the word might mean. Contextual clues can often give you all the information you need to decipher the meaning of an unfamiliar word. Even if you can't determine the meaning, you may be able to narrow down the possibilities enough to make a solid guess at the answer to the question.

⊘ PREFIXES

If you're having trouble with a word in the question or answer choices, try dissecting it. Take advantage of every clue that the word might include. Prefixes can be a huge help. Usually, they allow you to determine a basic meaning. *Pre-* means before, *post-* means after, *pro-* is positive, *de-* is negative. From prefixes, you can get an idea of the general meaning of the word and try to put it into context.

⊘ HEDGE WORDS

Watch out for critical hedge words, such as *likely, may, can, sometimes, often, almost, mostly, usually, generally, rarely,* and *sometimes*. Question writers insert these hedge phrases to cover every possibility. Often an answer choice will be wrong simply because it leaves no room for exception. Be on guard for answer choices that have definitive words such as *exactly* and *always*.

⊘ SWITCHBACK WORDS

Stay alert for *switchbacks*. These are the words and phrases frequently used to alert you to shifts in thought. The most common switchback words are *but, although,* and *however*. Others include *nevertheless, on the other hand, even though, while, in spite of, despite,* and *regardless of*. Switchback words are important to catch because they can change the direction of the question or an answer choice.

10

⊘ FACE VALUE

When in doubt, use common sense. Accept the situation in the problem at face value. Don't read too much into it. These problems will not require you to make wild assumptions. If you have to go beyond creativity and warp time or space in order to have an answer choice fit the question, then you should move on and consider the other answer choices. These are normal problems rooted in reality. The applicable relationship or explanation may not be readily apparent, but it is there for you to figure out. Use your common sense to interpret anything that isn't clear.

Answer Choice Strategies

⊘ ANSWER SELECTION

The most thorough way to pick an answer choice is to identify and eliminate wrong answers until only one is left, then confirm it is the correct answer. Sometimes an answer choice may immediately seem right, but be careful. The test writers will usually put more than one reasonable answer choice on each question, so take a second to read all of them and make sure that the other choices are not equally obvious. As long as you have time left, it is better to read every answer choice than to pick the first one that looks right without checking the others.

⊘ ANSWER CHOICE FAMILIES

An answer choice family consists of two (in rare cases, three) answer choices that are very similar in construction and cannot all be true at the same time. If you see two answer choices that are direct opposites or parallels, one of them is usually the correct answer. For instance, if one answer choice says that quantity x increases and another either says that quantity x decreases (opposite) or says that quantity y increases (parallel), then those answer choices would fall into the same family. An answer choice that doesn't match the construction of the answer choice family is more likely to be incorrect. Most questions will not have answer choice families, but when they do appear, you should be prepared to recognize them.

⊘ ELIMINATE ANSWERS

Eliminate answer choices as soon as you realize they are wrong, but make sure you consider all possibilities. If you are eliminating answer choices and realize that the last one you are left with is also wrong, don't panic. Start over and consider each choice again. There may be something you missed the first time that you will realize on the second pass.

⊘ AVOID FACT TRAPS

Don't be distracted by an answer choice that is factually true but doesn't answer the question. You are looking for the choice that answers the question. Stay focused on what the question is asking for so you don't accidentally pick an answer that is true but incorrect. Always go back to the question and make sure the answer choice you've selected actually answers the question and is not merely a true statement.

⊘ EXTREME STATEMENTS

In general, you should avoid answers that put forth extreme actions as standard practice or proclaim controversial ideas as established fact. An answer choice that states the "process should be used in certain situations, if…" is much more likely to be correct than one that states the "process should be discontinued completely." The first is a calm rational statement and doesn't even make a definitive, uncompromising stance, using a hedge word *if* to provide wiggle room, whereas the second choice is far more extreme.

⊘ Benchmark

As you read through the answer choices and you come across one that seems to answer the question well, mentally select that answer choice. This is not your final answer, but it's the one that will help you evaluate the other answer choices. The one that you selected is your benchmark or standard for judging each of the other answer choices. Every other answer choice must be compared to your benchmark. That choice is correct until proven otherwise by another answer choice beating it. If you find a better answer, then that one becomes your new benchmark. Once you've decided that no other choice answers the question as well as your benchmark, you have your final answer.

⊘ Predict the Answer

Before you even start looking at the answer choices, it is often best to try to predict the answer. When you come up with the answer on your own, it is easier to avoid distractions and traps because you will know exactly what to look for. The right answer choice is unlikely to be word-for-word what you came up with, but it should be a close match. Even if you are confident that you have the right answer, you should still take the time to read each option before moving on.

General Strategies

⊘ Tough Questions

If you are stumped on a problem or it appears too hard or too difficult, don't waste time. Move on! Remember though, if you can quickly check for obviously incorrect answer choices, your chances of guessing correctly are greatly improved. Before you completely give up, at least try to knock out a couple of possible answers. Eliminate what you can and then guess at the remaining answer choices before moving on.

⊘ Check Your Work

Since you will probably not know every term listed and the answer to every question, it is important that you get credit for the ones that you do know. Don't miss any questions through careless mistakes. If at all possible, try to take a second to look back over your answer selection and make sure you've selected the correct answer choice and haven't made a costly careless mistake (such as marking an answer choice that you didn't mean to mark). This quick double check should more than pay for itself in caught mistakes for the time it costs.

⊘ Pace Yourself

It's easy to be overwhelmed when you're looking at a page full of questions; your mind is confused and full of random thoughts, and the clock is ticking down faster than you would like. Calm down and maintain the pace that you have set for yourself. Especially as you get down to the last few minutes of the test, don't let the small numbers on the clock make you panic. As long as you are on track by monitoring your pace, you are guaranteed to have time for each question.

⊘ Don't Rush

It is very easy to make errors when you are in a hurry. Maintaining a fast pace in answering questions is pointless if it makes you miss questions that you would have gotten right otherwise. Test writers like to include distracting information and wrong answers that seem right. Taking a little extra time to avoid careless mistakes can make all the difference in your test score. Find a pace that allows you to be confident in the answers that you select.

⊘ Keep Moving

Panicking will not help you pass the test, so do your best to stay calm and keep moving. Taking deep breaths and going through the answer elimination steps you practiced can help to break through a stress barrier and keep your pace.

Final Notes

The combination of a solid foundation of content knowledge and the confidence that comes from practicing your plan for applying that knowledge is the key to maximizing your performance on test day. As your foundation of content knowledge is built up and strengthened, you'll find that the strategies included in this chapter become more and more effective in helping you quickly sift through the distractions and traps of the test to isolate the correct answer.

Now that you're preparing to move forward into the test content chapters of this book, be sure to keep your goal in mind. As you read, think about how you will be able to apply this information on the test. If you've already seen sample questions for the test and you have an idea of the question format and style, try to come up with questions of your own that you can answer based on what you're reading. This will give you valuable practice applying your knowledge in the same ways you can expect to on test day.

Good luck and good studying!

14

Cardiac, Vascular, and Pulmonary Systems

Cardiac Physical Therapy Data Collection

ANATOMY OF THE HEART

The heart consists of four chambers responsible for holding blood during the cycles of pumping. In the order of blood circulation, the **chambers** include the following:

- **Right atrium** (right upper): Receives deoxygenated blood from the venous system via major veins called the superior vena cava (from the head, neck, and upper body) and the inferior vena cava (from the internal organs and lower body).
- **Right ventricle** (right lower): Receives blood from the right atrium, and sends it to the lungs (pulmonary circulation) via the pulmonary artery.
- **Left atrium** (left upper): Receives oxygenated blood from the lungs via the pulmonary veins.
- **Left ventricle** (left lower): Receives blood from the left atrium, and pumps it into systemic circulation via the ascending and descending portions of the largest artery, the aorta.

Valves between chambers prevent backflow of blood between chambers or between the chambers and blood vessels:

- **Tricuspid valve**: Located between the right atrium and ventricle
- **Pulmonary valve**: Located between the right ventricle and pulmonary artery
- **Mitral valve**: Located between the left atrium and ventricle
- **Aortic valve**: Located between the left ventricle and aorta

15

The **arteries** that supply blood to the muscles of the heart are the coronary arteries.

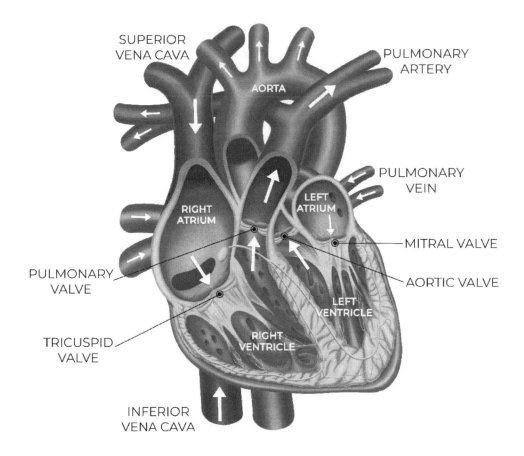

HEART TISSUES AND THEIR FUNCTIONS

The types of heart tissues are as follows:

- **Pericardium**: The double-walled sac enclosing the heart, with a tough outer surface (fibrous pericardium) and inner serous membrane (serous pericardium); protects against infection and trauma.
- **Epicardium**: The outermost layer of the cardiac wall and the visceral layer of the serous pericardium; protects against infection and trauma.
- **Myocardium**: The central, thick muscular layer of heart tissue, which provides pumping power to ventricles.

- **Endocardium**: The thin tissue layer lining many structures within the heart, including the chambers and valves.
- **Chordae tendineae and associated papillary muscles**: Tendons and muscles that prevent the eversion (turning inside out) of valves during ventricular systole.

Cardiac Cycle

A cardiac cycle is the time between heart contractions. Each heart chamber has a period of filling or relaxation, called **diastole**, followed by a period of contraction, called **systole**. The right side of the heart receives blood from the higher-pressure superior and inferior venae cavae essentially passively, whereas the left side of the heart requires sufficient high-pressure pumping power to circulate blood. Each atrium has a phase of atrial diastole followed by atrial systole. During atrial systole, about 70% of the blood empties into the corresponding ventricle, initially because of the pressure differential. The rest is then expelled through contraction or atrial kick. Ventricular diastole is the ventricular filling, which begins passively, and is followed by stretching of the ventricular walls during the corresponding atrial contraction. Ventricular systole or contraction follows, creating pressure before rapid ejection of the blood. The blood expelled from the ventricle is called the ejection fraction, typically about 60% for the left ventricle.

Cardiac Output

Cardiac output (CO) is the amount of blood pumped through the ventricles during a specified period. Normal cardiac output is about 5 liters per minutes at rest for an adult. Under exercise or stress, this volume may multiply 3 or 4 times with concomitant changes in the heart rate (HR) and stroke volume (SV). The basic formulation for calculating cardiac output is the heart rate (HR) per minute multiplied by the stroke volume (SR), which is the amount of blood pumped through the ventricles with each contraction. The stroke volume is controlled by preload, afterload, and contractibility.

$$\text{CO}\left(\frac{\text{mL}}{\text{min}}\right) = \text{HR}\left(\frac{\text{beats}}{\text{min}}\right) \times \text{SV (mL)}$$

The heart rate is controlled by the autonomic nervous system. Normally, if the heart rate decreases, stroke volume increases to compensate. The exception to this would be cardiomyopathies, so bradycardia results in a sharp decline in cardiac output.

Cardiac Conduction System

The heart has three characteristics directly related to electrical impulses:

- **Automaticity**: The ability to initiate internal electrical impulses
- **Excitability**: The capability to respond to electrical stimuli
- **Conductivity**: The transmission of electrical impulses between cells in the heart

The heart also has **contractility**, the capacity to stretch and recoil as a unit, and **rhythmicity**, the ability to repeat this sequence with regularity. The cardiac conduction system facilitates contraction and pumping of blood and influences heart rate. It is controlled intrinsically by several areas that transmit electrical impulses. In order, they are the sinoatrial (SA) node in the right atrium near the entrance of the superior vena cava, the atrioventricular (AV) node in the floor of the right atrium, the bundle of His between the two ventricles, branches from the bundle of His called the right and left bundle branches, and, ultimately, the Purkinje fibers. Successful conduction stimulates the myocardium, initiating ventricular contraction. There are also extrinsic controls, primarily the vagus nerve of the parasympathetic system and the upper thoracic nerves of the

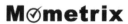

sympathetic branches of the autonomic nervous system, which decelerate or accelerate heart rate respectively.

IMPACT OF HORMONES ON CARDIAC FUNCTION

A number of bodily hormones affect cardiac function, either by influencing blood volume, causing vasoconstriction, or triggering vasodilation. In the atria of the heart, there are **atrial natriuretic peptides** that can be stimulated by increased atrial stretch, resulting in lower blood volume by stimulating diuresis. Blood volume can be increased by the hormone **aldosterone**, which is stimulated when there is hypovolemia or decreased renal perfusion. Vasoconstriction or the narrowing of blood vessels, which reduces blood flow and increases blood pressure, can be induced by **norepinephrine** during stress or exercise, or angiotensin or **vasopressin** in response to decreased arterial pressure. Hormones that can cause vasodilation or widening of blood vessels include **epinephrine** in response to stress or exercise, and **bradykinin** and **histamine** in response to tissue damage.

PROCESS OF SYSTEMIC CIRCULATION

Systemic circulation is the flow of blood through the body. It is initiated when oxygenated blood is ejected from the left ventricle during systole into the large artery, the aorta. The aorta diverges into smaller arteries, then narrower arterioles, and eventually even narrower capillaries. There is an exchange of gases at the capillary level, in which oxygen (O_2) is distributed to the surrounding tissues and carbon dioxide (CO_2) is taken in. The deoxygenated blood travels from the capillaries into larger venules, then wider veins, and ultimately the venae cavae into the heart. The systemic circulation on the venous side is facilitated by muscular contractions and pressures, as well as unidirectional valves that prevent blood backflow.

LAYERS OF BLOOD VESSELS

All blood vessels have three layers. The innermost layer is called the **tunica intima**, which is composed of endothelial cells over a basement membrane and provides a smooth surface for laminar blood flow. The middle layer is termed the **tunica media**, consisting of smooth muscle cells and elastic connective tissue. The tunica media is also innervated by sympathetic nerves and is the layer responsible for constriction and dilation of the vessel to control blood pressure. The outermost layer is known as the **tunica externa**. This section is made up of collagen fibers (connective tissue), lymph vessels, and other blood vessels that supply it with nutrients.

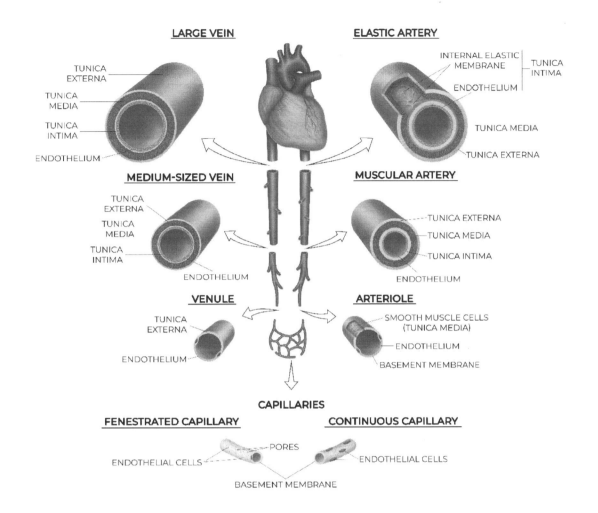

TYPES OF BLOOD VESSELS

The three types of blood vessels are arteries, veins, and capillaries.

- All **arteries** have a thick middle or tunica media layer that permits them to adjust to pressure changes from the heart. There are large, relatively elastic arteries, such as the aorta, its large branches, and the pulmonary artery; medium-sized ones like the coronary arteries, which are more muscular; and small arteries and arterioles. Most arteries carry oxygenated blood from the heart.
- **Veins** come in a range of diameters from small to large. They have a thin tunica media layer but a thick outer tunica externa. Veins carry deoxygenated blood to the heart and have valves that thwart backflow of blood and aid in the venous return.
- **Capillaries** are the narrowest type of blood vessel, found at the convergence between the arterial and venous systems. Gases, as well as blood cells and fluids, are exchanged at the capillary level. The configuration of each capillary bed or mass is dependent on the circulatory requirements in the area.

TYPES OF BLOOD CELLS

Blood cells fall into the following three categories:

- **Erythrocytes** are red blood cells (RBCs) that contain hemoglobin. Hemoglobin consists of four protein chains attached to pigment complexes containing iron. It transports oxygen to tissues through the attachment of oxygen to the iron, forming oxyhemoglobin.
- **Leukocytes** are white blood cells (WBCs). There are five varieties of leukocytes, all of which play some role in immune defense and fighting off infection. WBCs include neutrophils, basophils, eosinophils, lymphocytes, and monocytes.
- The third type of blood cell is a **platelet** or thrombocyte, which is involved in clot formation.

FUNCTIONS OF BLOOD

Blood is involved in oxygen and carbon dioxide transport through hemoglobin binds. Nutrients and metabolites are transported by binding to plasma proteins. The plasma portion of blood carries hormones throughout the body, waste products to the liver and kidneys, and cells and other molecules involved in the immune response to infection sites. Many of the blood's functions are related to regulation of bodily functions. These include maintenance of fluid balance through adjustment of blood volume, optimal body temperature via vasoconstriction or dilation, and acid-base balance. Blood also preserves hemostasis by clotting and halting bleeding and hemorrhaging.

PATIENT HISTORY

In terms of cardiac evaluation, the patient history should address whether the patient has experienced any chest pain, cardiac risk factors, palpitations (fast or irregular heartbeats), prior myocardial infarction (MI) or cardiac-related tests, a family history of cardiac disease, or a history of dizziness or fainting. The history should also include the related medical treatment administered and its effect. Chest pain or angina should be described in terms of its location and radiation, its frequency, the quality of the pain (for example crushing, numbing, or burning), what the patient is describing as chest pain (for example, shortness of breath, dizziness, jaw pain, etc.), and the factors that precipitate, aggravate, and alleviate the pain. Chest pain generally indicates lack of blood to the heart.

CARDIAC RISK FACTORS

Cardiac risk factors should be addressed in the patient's history. The main independent risk factors for cardiac problems are smoking, hypertension, diabetes mellitus, aging, and a poor cholesterol profile (high total cholesterol and high LDL and/or low HDL). Other factors that can predispose individuals to cardiac issues should also be included in the history and include physical inactivity; a body mass index of > 30 kg/m^2; obesity, particularly abdominal (high waist-hip ratio, waist > 40" for men and > 35" for women); family history of early heart disease; psychosocial issues; and ethnic background. There are a number of substances in the blood which, when elevated, may also be indicative of cardiac risk. These include triglycerides, homocysteine, lipoprotein (a), or inflammatory markers. The presence of small LDL particles, C-reactive protein (CRP), or fibrinogen can also indicate cardiac risk.

CARDIAC ASSESSMENT

Data collection of the heart includes collection of vital signs, heart and lung sounds, skin evaluation, radial, popliteal, and pedal pulses, circulation and sensation of extremities, and auscultation of the aorta, renal, iliac, and femoral arteries for bruits. Blood should be taken for a lipid profile and electrolytes. The patient must be helped to modify risk factors such as hypertension, smoking, diabetes, obesity, hyperlipidemia, inactivity, and stress.

PALPATION OF THE PULSE

Palpation is a method of clinical evaluation that uses gentle pressure with the fingers. In terms of cardiac evaluation, it is used to measure the person's pulse and to check extremities for pitting edema. Some of the more common spots for checking the pulse are the radial artery in the wrist, the carotid artery in the neck, or the brachial artery at the bend of the arm (commonly used in infants). Pulses give an indication of circulation quality, heart rate (HR), and rhythm. Pulse amplitude is classified on a scale from 0 to 4+.

- 0 indicates no pulse or circulation.
- 1+ designates a diminished pulse (from factors like increased vascular resistance and lowered stroke volume and ejection fraction).
- 2+ is a normal resting pulse.
- 3+ indicates a moderately increased pulse.
- 4+ means a markedly increased or bounding pulse.

The latter two are associated with varying degrees of increased stroke volume and ejection fraction. Possible pulse abnormalities include pulsus alternans (alternating strong and weak pulses indicative of left ventricular failure), pulsus paradoxus (weak pulse and low blood pressure during inspiration associated with a number of cardiopulmonary problems), and bigeminal pulses (every other pulse weak and premature due to pre-ventricular contractions).

PALPATION FOR PITTING EDEMA

Palpation is also used during a physical examination as part of a cardiac evaluation to check the extremities bilaterally for pitting edema. Edema is swelling due to a buildup of excess fluid which, among other things, could be due to circulation or pumping problems. The pitting edema scale ranges from 1+ to 4+ as follows:

- 1+: **Trace**; scarcely perceptible depression observed with palpation.
- 2+: **Mild**; an easily identified depression (EID) up to 4 mm, where the skin rebounds in less than 15 seconds.
- 3+: **Moderate**; a 4-8 mm EID, which rebounds in 15-30 seconds.
- 4+: **Severe**; an EID greater than 8 mm, with a rebound that takes more than 30 seconds.

BLOOD PRESSURE

Blood pressure (BP), a vital sign, should be taken as part of a physical examination. BP measurement indirectly quantifies the force against arterial walls during the phases of ventricular systole (pumping) and diastole (filling). A cuff with an inflatable bladder and pressure gauge, called a sphygmomanometer, is used. The patient should be seated with their arm resting at heart level. At the outset, readings should be taken on both arms and the arm with higher readings should be used. At least two readings separated by as much time as possible should be taken. The appropriate size cuff is wrapped around the arm approximately 1 inch above the antecubital crease. The bladder is inflated with the attached bulb to a pressure 20-40 mmHg above the systolic pressure, which is indicated when a radial pulse (palpated simultaneously) disappears. The bladder is then deflated at a rate of 3 mmHg/second while the clinician uses a stethoscope to listen for characteristic Korotkoff sounds indicating first systolic (initial faint tapping) and then diastolic pressure (muffled or absent). BP can also be taken on the thigh with auscultation at the popliteal artery at the knee.

KOROTKOFF SOUNDS

Korotkoff sounds are characteristic sounds heard with a stethoscope while deflating the sphygmomanometer around 2-3 mmHg per second. A phase one Korotkoff sound, which is a faint

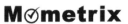

tapping noise that gets louder, should be heard first. This indicates the systolic pressure or point at which the blood starts to flow through the compressed artery. As the bladder is deflated more, a phase two swishing sound is heard, followed by phase three louder tapping. As deflation continues, at some point, the sounds become more muffled (phase four). In children younger than 13 years of age or adults who are exercising, pregnant, or hyperthyroid, this muffling indicates the diastolic pressure. However, for normal resting adults, the diastolic pressure is not reached until the Korotkoff sounds disappear (phase five), which is generally 5-10 mmHg lower than phase four.

NORMAL BLOOD PRESSURE RANGES

Blood pressure (BP) is always expressed as a ratio of two numbers, the first of which is the systolic pressure and the second being the diastolic pressure. Normal values depend on age.

Normal blood pressure values are as follows:

- At age 8: Systolic 85-115 mmHg, diastolic 55-75 mmHg
- At age 12: Systolic 95-120 mmHg, diastolic 60-80 mmHg
- Adults: Systolic <120 mmHg, diastolic <80 mmHg

For adults, prehypertension and hypertension (high blood pressure indicative of arterial disease) are defined as:

- **Prehypertension**: Systolic 120-129 mmHg; diastolic <80 mmHg
- **Stage 1 hypertension**: Systolic 130-139 mmHg; diastolic 80-89 mmHg
- **Stage 2 hypertension**: Systolic ≥140 mmHg; diastolic ≥90 mmHg

Individuals who are exercising are expected to have increased systolic pressure of 5-12 mmHg per MET (metabolic equivalent) in workload while their diastolic readings should remain within 10 mmHg of their normal value.

AUSCULTATION OF HEART SOUNDS

Auscultation of heart sounds can help to diagnose different cardiac disorders. Areas to auscultate include the aortic area, pulmonary area, Erb's point, tricuspid area, and the apical area. The **normal heart sounds** represent closing of the valves.

- The **first heart sound** (S1) "lub" is closure of the mitral and tricuspid valves (heard at apex/left ventricular area of the heart).
- The **second heart sound** (S2) "dub" is closure of the aortic and pulmonic valves (heard at the base of the heart). There may be a slight splitting of the S2.

The time between S1 and S2 is systole and the time between S2 and the next S1 is diastole. Systole and diastole should be silent although ventricular disease can cause gallops, snaps, or clicks and stenosis of the valves or failure of the valves to close can cause murmurs. Pericarditis may cause a friction rub.

Additional heart sounds:

- **Gallop rhythms**: S3 commonly occurs after S2 in children and young adults but may indicate heart failure or left ventricular failure in older adults (when heard with patient lying on left side). S4 occurs before S1, during the contracting of the atria when there is ventricular hypertrophy, found in coronary artery disease, hypertension, or aortic valve stenosis.

- **Opening snap**: Unusual high-pitched sound occurring after S2 with stenosis of mitral valve from rheumatic heart disease
- **Ejection click**: Brief high-pitched sound after S1; aortic stenosis
- **Friction rub**: Harsh, grating holosystolic sound; pericarditis
- **Murmur**: Sound caused by turbulent blood flow from stenotic or malfunctioning valves, congenital defects, or increased blood flow. Murmurs are characterized by location, timing in the cardiac cycle, intensity (rated from Grade I to Grade VI), pitch (low to high-pitched), quality (rumbling, whistling, blowing) and radiation (to the carotids, axilla, neck, shoulder, or back).

ELECTROCARDIOGRAM

The electrocardiogram records and shows a graphic display of the electrical activity of the heart through a number of different waveforms, complexes, and intervals:

- **P wave**: Start of electrical impulse in the sinus node and spreading through the atria, muscle depolarization
- **QRS complex**: Ventricular muscle depolarization and atrial repolarization
- **T wave**: Ventricular muscle repolarization (resting state) as cells regain negative charge
- **U wave**: Repolarization of the Purkinje fibers

A modified lead II ECG is often used to monitor basic heart rhythms and dysrhythmias:

- Typical placement of leads for 2-lead ECG is 3-5 cm inferior to the right clavicle and left lower ribcage. Typical placement for a 3-lead ECG is (RA) right arm near shoulder, (LA) V_5 position over 5th intercostal space, and (LL) left upper leg near groin.

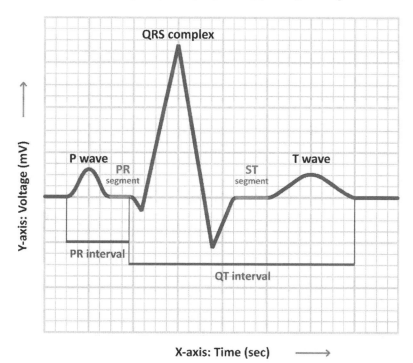

In a hospital, a patient may be hooked up to three to five leads and continuously monitored through telemetry being monitored by a trained clinician or a patient monitor within the patient's room (used in acute care units). In the case of telemetry, data is recorded on tape or by telemetric ECG monitoring, which sends signals in real-time to a monitor for observation.

CARDIAC-RELATED LABORATORY TESTING
COMPLETE BLOOD CELL COUNT (CBC)

A complete blood cell count (CBC) is an important evaluation tool for an individual's cardiac and vascular systems. It consists of several results, including the following:

- RBC count
- WBC count
- WBC differential
- Hematocrit
- Hemoglobin
- Platelet

WHITE BLOOD CELL (WBC) COUNT AND DIFFERENTIAL

White blood cell (leukocyte) count is used as an indicator of bacterial and viral infection. WBC count is reported as the total number of all white blood cells.

- Normal WBC for adults: 4,800-10,000
- Acute infection: 10,000+; 30,000 indicates a severe infection
- Viral infection: 4,000 and below

The **differential** provides the percentage of each different type of leukocyte. An increase in the white blood cell count is usually related to an increase in one type, and often an increase in immature neutrophils (bands), referred to as a "shift to the left," is an indication of an infectious process:

- Normal immature neutrophils (bands): 1-3%, increases with infection
- Normal segmented neutrophils (segs) for adults: 50-62%, increases with acute, localized, or systemic bacterial infections
- Normal eosinophils: 0-3%, decreases with stress and acute infection
- Normal basophils: 0-1%, decreases during acute stage of infection
- Normal lymphocytes: 25-40%, increases in some viral and bacterial infections
- Normal monocytes: 3-7%, increases during recovery stage of acute infection

RED BLOOD CELLS

Red blood cells (RBCs or erythrocytes) are biconcave disks that contain **hemoglobin** (95% of mass), which carries oxygen throughout the body. The heme portion of the cell contains **iron**, which binds to the oxygen. RBCs live about 120 days, after which they are destroyed and their hemoglobin is recycled or excreted. Normal values of **red blood cell count** vary by gender:

- Males >18 years: 4.7-6.1 million per mm^3
- Females >18 years: 4.2-5.4 million per mm^3

The most common **disorders of RBCs** are those that interfere with production, leading to various types of **anemia**:

- Blood loss
- Hemolysis
- Bone marrow failure

The **morphology** of RBCs may vary depending upon the type of anemia:

- Size: Normocytes, microcytes, macrocytes
- Shape: Spherocytes (round), poikilocytes (irregular), drepanocytes (sickled)
- Color (reflecting concentration of hemoglobin): Normochromic, hypochromic

LABORATORY TESTS

A number of different tests are used to evaluate the condition and production of red blood cells in addition to the red blood cell count.

Hemoglobin: Carries oxygen and is decreased in anemia and increased in polycythemia. Normal values:

- Males >18 years: 14.0-17.46 g/dL
- Females >18 years: 12.0-16.0 g/dL

Hematocrit: Indicates the proportion of RBCs in a liter of blood (usually about 3 times the hemoglobin number). Normal values:

- Males >18 years: 40-50%
- Females >18 years: 35-45%

Mean corpuscular volume (MCV): Indicates the size of RBCs and can differentiate types of anemia. For adults, <80 is microcytic and >100 is macrocytic. Normal values:

- Males >18 years: 84-96 μm^3
- Females >18 years: 76-96 μm^3

Reticulocyte count: Measures marrow production and should rise with anemia. Normal values: 0.5-1.5% of total RBCs.

ERYTHROCYTE SEDIMENTATION RATE (ESR)

Erythrocyte sedimentation rate (sed rate) measures the distance erythrocytes fall in a vertical tube of anticoagulated blood in one hour. Because fibrinogen, which increases in response to infection, also increases the rate of the fall, the sed rate can be used as a non-specific test for inflammation when infection is suspected. The sed rate is sensitive to osteomyelitis and may be used to monitor treatment response. Values vary according to gender and age:

- <50: Males 0-15 mm/hr; females 0-20 mm/hr
- >50: Males 0-20 mm/hr; females 0-30 mm/hr

COAGULATION PROFILE

The coagulation profile measures clotting mechanisms, identifies clotting disorders, screens preoperative patients, and diagnoses excessive bruising and bleeding. Values vary depending on lab:

- Prothrombin time (PT): 10-14 seconds
  - Increases with anticoagulation therapy, vitamin K deficiency, decreased prothrombin, DIC, liver disease, and malignant neoplasm. Some drugs may shorten PT.
- Partial thromboplastin time (PTT): 25-35 seconds
  - Increases with hemophilia A and B, von Willebrand disease, vitamin deficiency, lupus, DIC, and liver disease.
- Activated partial thromboplastin time (aPTT): 21-35 seconds
  - Similar to PTT, but decreases in extensive cancer, early DIC, and after acute hemorrhage. Used to monitor heparin dosage.
- Thrombin clotting time (TCT) or Thrombin time (TT): 7-12 seconds
  - Used most often to determine the dosage of heparin. Prolonged with multiple myeloma, abnormal fibrinogen, uremia, and liver disease.
- **Bleeding time**: 2-9.5 minutes
  - (Using the IVY method on the forearm) Increases with DIC, leukemia, renal failure, aplastic anemia, von Willebrand disease, some drugs, and alcohol.
- **Platelet count**: 150,000-400,000 per μL
  - Increased bleeding <50,000 (transfusion required) and increased clotting >750,000.

BLOOD LIPID TESTS

Blood lipid tests generally measure total cholesterol, low-density lipoproteins (LDLs), high-density lipoproteins (HDLs), and often triglycerides. All are some form of lipid, a fat constituent insoluble in water. High total cholesterol puts an individual at risk for atherosclerosis (blood flow obstruction due to plaques) and ischemic heart disease. LDLs comprise the portion that sticks to the inner walls of blood vessels; therefore, a high LDL level is also associated with a propensity toward coronary artery disease (CAD). The larger HDLs do not adhere to internal walls but flow freely and actually lower risk of CAD. High triglyceride levels have also been associated with CAD.

Current normal values are:

- **Total cholesterol**: < 200 mg/dL (> 240 mg/dL considered high)
- **LDLs**: < 100 mg/dL
- **HDLs**: > 33 mg/dL for males; > 43 mg/dl for females

The ratio of total cholesterol to HDL should be between three and five.

C-REACTIVE PROTEIN (CRP)

C-reactive protein is an acute-phase reactant produced by the liver in response to an inflammatory response that causes neutrophils, granulocytes, and macrophages to secrete cytokines. Thus, levels of C-reactive protein rise when there is inflammation or infection. It is helpful to measure the response to treatment for pyoderma gangrenosum ulcers:

- Normal values: 2.6-7.6 μg/dL

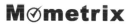

CARDIAC BIOCHEMICAL MARKERS

Creatine kinase (CK) and CK-MB levels are evaluated every 6–8 hours in a suspected myocardial injury. Total CK and CK-MB (specific to cardiac cells) initially rise within the first 4–6 hours of an MI. A normal range would be 30 IU/L to 180 IU/L for CK and CK-MB totaling 0–5% of the CK level.

Assuming no further damage is sustained, peak levels (in excess of 6 times the normal range) are reached 12–24 hours after the injury. CK levels will return to normal within 3–4 days of the event. Small spikes in CK level might also occur following invasive cardiac procedures.

Troponin, which is found in cardiac and skeletal muscle, is a type of protein. Both troponin I and T (isolates of troponin) are found in the myocardium, but troponin T is also found in skeletal muscle, so it is less specific than troponin I. Troponin I, therefore, may be used to detect a myocardial infarction after non-cardiac surgery and to detect acute coronary syndrome. Troponin is released into the bloodstream when injury to the tissue (such as the myocardium) occurs and causes damage to the cell membranes, as occurs with myocardial injury.

- **Troponin I** (<0.05 ng/mL): Appears in 2-6 hours, peaks at 15-20 hours and returns to normal in 5-7 days. Exhibits a second but lower peak at 60-80 hours (biphasic).
- **Troponin T** (<0.2 ng/mL): Increases 2-6 hours after MI and stays elevated. Returns to normal in 7 days. (Less specific than troponin I)

NATRIURETIC PEPTIDES

The term natriuretic refers to the excretion of sodium. There are three natriuretic peptides termed atrial natriuretic peptide (ANP), brain natriuretic peptide (BNP), and C-natriuretic peptide (CNP). ANP and BNP have additional diuretic and vasodilation properties and are involved in homeostasis and blood pressure control; plasma levels of these two peptides are known to be elevated in individuals with heart failure. ANP and BNP are accrued in the right atrium and ventricles, respectively, and released when there is increased pressure in those areas. CNP is predominantly detected in the vasculature, but its role is somewhat unclear.

CARDIAC DIAGNOSTIC TOOLS

ECHOCARDIOGRAPHY

Echocardiography is a non-invasive ultrasound technology that is very useful for assessing and diagnosing anatomic heart abnormalities, blood flow, and valvular lesions:

- The **standard "2D Echo"** is used best for basic structural imaging, such as valvular lesions and assessment of pericardial disorders.
- The **transesophageal (TEE)** probe is an improved version of echocardiography, which allows better visualization of the left atrium and more precise evaluation of the valvular structure. TEE is also the best modality for evaluation of the thoracic aorta in the setting of suspected aortic dissection or aneurysm.
- **Doppler imaging** is used to measure blood flow, often in the context of velocity across a valve and a pressure gradient.
- **Bubble study** is an addition to echocardiography allowing the study to determine if there is right to left blood flow through a patent foramen ovale or a more distal intrapulmonary shunt of blood.

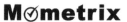

STRESS TESTING
INDICATIONS AND CONTRAINDICATIONS

Exercise, or stress testing, is the methodical and progressive use of some form of activity accompanied by concurrent ECG readings, blood pressure measurements, patient observation, and possibly pulmonary function analysis. It is most often used to diagnose the presence of coronary artery disease (CAD) and is also useful for predicting disease prognosis or severity, evaluating other cardiac problems like congestive heart failure or arrhythmias, and looking at functional capacity. Exercise testing can also be used to determine the person's safe heart rate range for activity. Exercise testing is contraindicated during acute illness and for cardiac patients who have had a myocardial infarction within the last 48 hours or who have unstable angina, acute pericarditis, ventricular or fast arrhythmias, untreated advanced heart block, or decompensated congestive heart failure.

PROCEDURE

Basic **cardiac stress testing** consists of exercise EKG testing (EET) and exercise imaging testing. The exercise imaging testing may be broken down into exercise, or "stress" echocardiography, and exercise myocardial perfusion imaging.

Exercise imaging testing is usually performed with echocardiography. Stress echocardiography is performed similarly to exercise EKG testing and also requires that the patient meet at least 85% maximum heart rate in order to attain optimum sensitivity and specificity. (The maximum heart rate formula is 220 minus the person's age.) Of note, chemicals may substitute for exercise during the "stress" portion of the test. This may be performed with dobutamine (beta-1-agonist: cannot be used after beta-blocker administration) or adenosine (causes diffuse coronary dilatation, leading to decreased perfusion pressure and unmasking of defects, and cannot be used with asthma). Stress imaging allows the study to determine the actual area of ischemia and whether or not this is a reversible defect. Additional information obtained during echocardiography is cardiac output and measurement of viability.

METABOLIC EQUIVALENTS AS THEY RELATE TO STRESS TESTING

Metabolic equivalents (METs) represent the ratio between an individual's metabolic rate while performing a particular activity compared to the metabolic rate while seated and resting (1 MET). The formula for calculation of 1 MET is:

$$1 \text{ MET} = 3.5 \text{ mL } O_2 \text{ uptake/kg per minute}$$

Most fit people can perform maximally around 8 METs. Some typical exercise test protocols push people to higher limits, around 13 METS, such as the Bruce Protocol for the treadmill and some bike ergometer protocols. METs are actually a measurement of oxygen consumption.

Walking pace (feet/minute) on a level surface is related to oxygen consumption. If a patient cannot sustain a particular walking pace for one minute, that pace is near their optimal METs or oxygen consumption. If they cannot maintain a particular walking pace for 10 minutes, then that rate is higher than their anaerobic threshold. A pace that can be sustained for 1-10 minutes should be used interspersed with rest for exercise testing.

CARDIAC CATHETERIZATION

Cardiac catheterization is an invasive process in which a flexible radiopaque catheter is delivered (usually through the radial or femoral vein or artery) into the heart for visualization of the anatomy. The procedure is used in conjunction with angiography, percutaneous transluminal coronary angioplasty (PTCA), cardiac muscles biopsies, and electrophysiologic studies (EPSs).

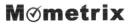

During angiography, a radiopaque contrast substance is injected via catheter to look at blood vessels or chambers. Various types include aortography of the aorta and its valve, coronary arteriography of the coronary arteries, ventriculography of either ventricle and the AV valves, and pulmonary angiography. EPSs involve insertion of an electrode catheter via the femoral vein into the right ventricle to look at electrical conduction in the heart. Cardiac catheters can be right-sided or left-sided and are typically inserted into the subclavian vein or femoral artery, respectively. The side for insertion is selected depending on the suspected cardiac issues on that side. A common use of right-sided catheterization is to monitor cardiac pressures in patients with heart failure. Patients that have undergone cardiac catheterization must remain on bed rest from four to six hours with the selected extremity immobilized.

Cardiac Disease/Conditions that Impact Effective Treatment

ACUTE CORONARY SYNDROME

Acute coronary syndrome (ACS) is the impairment of blood flow through the coronary arteries, leading to ischemia of the cardiac muscle. Angina frequently occurs in ACS, manifesting as crushing pain substernally, radiating down the left arm or both arms. However, in females, elderly, and diabetics, symptoms may appear less acute and include nausea, shortness of breath, fatigue, pain/weakness/numbness in arms, or no pain at all (silent ischemia). There are multiple **classifications of angina**:

- **Stable angina**: Exercise-induced, short lived, relieved by rest or nitroglycerin. Other precipitating events include decrease in environmental temperature, heavy eating, strong emotions (such as fright or anger), or exertion, including coitus.
- **Unstable angina** (preinfarction or crescendo angina): A change in the pattern of stable angina, characterized by an increase in pain, not responding to a single nitroglycerin or rest, and persisting for >5 minutes. May cause a change in EKG, or indicate rupture of an atherosclerotic plaque or the beginning of thrombus formation. Treat as a medical emergency, indicates impending MI.
- **Variant angina** (Prinzmetal's angina): Results from spasms of the coronary arteries. Associated with or without atherosclerotic plaques and is often related to smoking, alcohol, or illicit stimulants, but can occur cyclically and at rest. Elevation of ST segments usually occurs with variant angina. Treatment is nitroglycerin or calcium channel blockers.

MYOCARDIAL INFARCTIONS

Non–ST-segment elevation MI (NSTEMI): ST elevation on the electrocardiogram (ECG) occurs in response to myocardial damage resulting from infarction or severe ischemia. The absence of ST elevation may be diagnosed as unstable angina or NSTEMI, but cardiac enzyme levels increase with NSTEMI, indicating partial blockage of coronary arteries with some damage. Symptoms are consistent with unstable angina, with chest pain or tightness, pain radiating to the neck or arm, dyspnea, anxiety, weakness, dizziness, nausea, vomiting, and heartburn. Initial treatment may include nitroglycerin, β-blockers, antiplatelet agents, or antithrombotic agents. Ongoing treatment may include β-blockers, aspirin, statins, angiotensin-converting enzyme inhibitors, angiotensin-receptor blockers, and clopidogrel. Percutaneous coronary intervention is not recommended.

ST-segment elevation MI (STEMI): This more severe type of MI involves complete blockage of one or more coronary arteries with myocardial damage, resulting in ST elevation. Symptoms are those

29

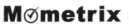
of acute MI. As necrosis occurs, Q waves often develop, indicating irreversible myocardial damage, which may result in death, so treatment involves immediate reperfusion before necrosis can occur.

> **Review Video: Myocardial Infarction**
> Visit mometrix.com/academy and enter code: 148923

CARDIAC RHYTHM AND CONDUCTION DISTURBANCES

There are four general categories of cardiac rhythm or conduction disturbances, and each has characteristic electrocardiographic (ECG) patterns. The four categories are as follows:

- **Atrial rhythm disturbances** include supraventricular tachycardia, atrial flutter, atrial fibrillation (AF), and premature atrial contractions.
- **Ventricular rhythm disturbances** include ventricular tachycardia (VT), multifocal VT (also called torsades de pointes), premature ventricular contractions, ventricular fibrillation, and idioventricular rhythm.
- **Junctional rhythm disturbances** include junctional escape rhythm and junctional tachycardia.
- **Atrioventricular (AV) blocks** include first-degree AV block, second-degree AV block type 1, second-degree AV block type II, and third-degree AV block (a complete heart attack).

ATRIAL RHYTHM DISTURBANCES

Atrial rhythm disturbances include the following:

- **Supraventricular tachycardia (SVT)** is characterized on an ECG by a regular rhythm and a high heart rate of 160-250 bpm. It is often due to rheumatoid heart disease (RHD), mitral valve prolapse, cor pulmonale, or digitalis toxicity. A physical therapist/physical therapist assistant should not treat such a patient until the supraventricular tachycardia subsides.

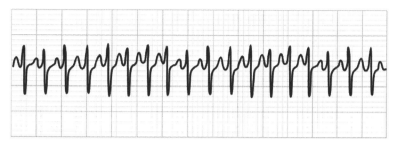

- **Atrial flutter** is distinguished by a high atrial rate of 250-350 bpm, with or without a regular rhythm. P waves are saw-toothed (referred to as F waves), QRS shape and duration (0.04-0.11 seconds) are usually normal, PR interval may be hard to calculate because of F waves, and the P:QRS ratio is 2:1 to 4:1. Symptoms include chest pain, dyspnea, and hypotension. It is generally due to coronary artery disease, mitral stenosis, or hypertension. The physical therapist should evaluate how well the patient tolerates atrial flutter before treating or having the physical therapist assistant treat the patient.

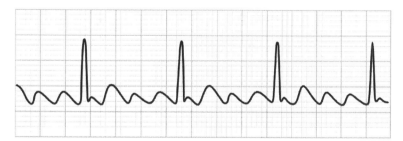

- **Atrial fibrillation (AFib)** is characterized by a very irregular pulse with atrial rate of 300-600 and ventricular rate of 120-200, shape and duration (0.04-0.11 seconds) of QRS is usually normal. Fibrillatory (F) waves are seen instead of P waves. The PR interval cannot be measured and the P:QRS ratio is highly variable. It can occur in association with many types of cardiac disease, including CHF, CAD, RHD, cor pulmonale, and hypertension. Chronic cases can be treated carefully, but new ones should be attended to medically first.

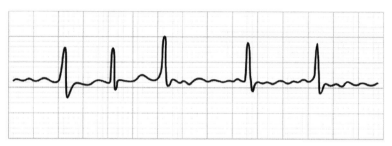

- **Premature atrial contractions** are seen as a normal heart rate (60-100 bpm) that displays irregular rhythm, sometimes sporadic. They can be attributed simply to lifestyle issues, like caffeine ingestion, but may also indicate CAD, CHF, or electrolyte imbalance—the patient may be asymptomatic. These contractions can precede development of AFib.

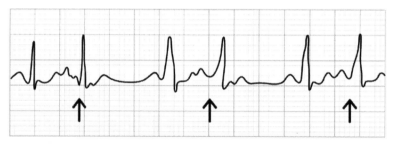

> **Review Video: <u>EKG Interpretation: Afib and Aflutter</u>**
> Visit mometrix.com/academy and enter code: 263842

VENTRICULAR RHYTHM DISTURBANCES

Ventricular rhythm disturbances include the following:

- **Premature ventricular contractions (PVCs)** are those in which the impulse begins in the ventricles and conducts through them prior to the next sinus impulse. The ectopic QRS complexes may vary in shape, depending upon whether there is one site (unifocal) or more (multifocal) that stimulates the ectopic beats. PVCs usually cause no morbidity unless there is underlying cardiac disease or an acute MI. PVCs are characterized by an irregular heartbeat, QRS that is ≥0.12 seconds and oddly shaped. They can occur in normal individuals subsequent to things like caffeine use but are also associated with CAD, MI, and other cardiac diseases. Treatment depends on the rate of occurrence.

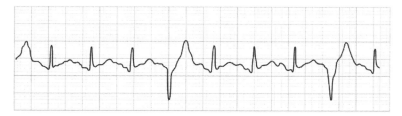

- **Ventricular tachycardia (VT)** is greater than 3 PVCs in a row with a ventricular rate of 100-200 beats per minute. A detectable rate is usually regular and the QRS complex is ≥0.12 seconds and is usually abnormally shaped. The P wave may be undetectable with an irregular PR interval if P wave is present. The usual cause is coronary artery disease subsequent to acute MI. Patients require immediate medical attention, not physical therapy. Multifocal VT, or torsades de pointes, is similar on an ECG except that the rate is higher, > 150 bpm. It is usually induced by the use of antiarrhythmic drugs, MI, low electrolyte levels of potassium or magnesium, or hypothermia. Again, medical attention, not physical therapy, is indicated.

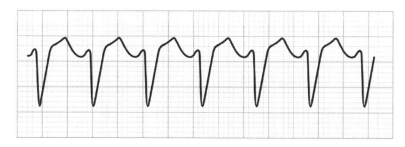

- **Ventricular fibrillation (VFib)** is a rapid, very irregular ventricular rate >300 beats per minute with no atrial activity observable on the ECG, caused by disorganized electrical activity in the ventricles. The QRS complex is not recognizable as ECG shows irregular undulations. This is a medical emergency and requires immediate medical attention, not physical therapy.

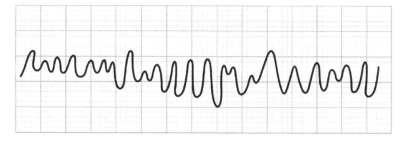

- **Idioventricular rhythm** is regular but in the range of 20-40 bpm, indicating advanced cardiac disease that generally should be left untreated.

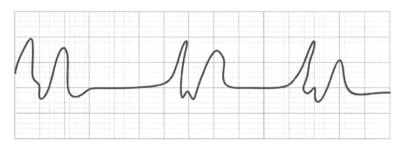

- **Agonal rhythm** is an irregular rhythm with an extremely low rate of < 20 bpm and no P wave, indicating the patient is close to death and should not be treated.

> **Review Video: EKG Interpretation: Ventricular Arrythmias**
> Visit mometrix.com/academy and enter code: 933152

JUNCTIONAL RHYTHM DISTURBANCES

Junctional rhythms occur when the AV node becomes the pacemaker of the heart. This can happen because the sinus node is depressed from increased vagal tone or a block at the AV node prevents sinus node impulses from being transmitted. While the sinus node normally sends impulses 60-100 beats per minute, the AV node junction usually sends impulses at 40-60 beats per minute. The QRS complex is of usual shape and duration (0.04-0.11 seconds). The P wave may be inverted and may be absent, hidden or after the QRS. If the P wave precedes the QRS, the PR interval is <0.12 seconds. The P:QRS ratio is <1:1 or 1:1. The junctional escape rhythm is a protective mechanism preventing asystole with failure of the sinus node. An **accelerated junctional rhythm** is similar, but the heart rate is 60-100. **Junctional tachycardia** occurs with heart rate of >100.

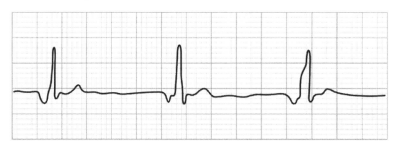

ATRIOVENTRICULAR (AV) BLOCKS

Atrioventricular (AV) blocks include the following:

- **First-degree AV blocks** are characterized on an ECG by a normal rhythm and rate but a prolonged PR interval greater than 0.2 seconds. They are usually seen in elderly patients with heart disease, acute myocarditis, or during acute myocardial infarction. The underlying heart disease really determines how to treat these patients, and new blockage should be monitored for progression.

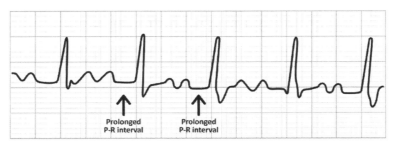

- **Second-degree AV blocks** are characterized on the ECG by an irregular rhythm and an atrial rate higher than the ventricular one. There are two types.
  - *Mobitz type I block (Wenckebach)* occurs when each atrial impulse in a group of beats is conducted at a lengthened interval until one fails to conduct (the PR interval progressively increases), so there are more P waves than QRS complexes, but the QRS complex is usually of normal shape and duration. Patients with a type I block are usually asymptomatic.

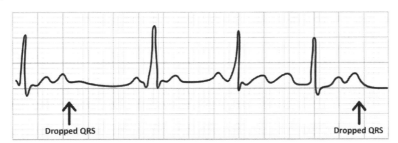

  - In *Mobitz type II*, only some of the atrial impulses are conducted unpredictably through the AV node to the ventricles, and the block always occurs below the AV node in the bundle of His, the bundle branches, or the Purkinje fibers. The PR intervals are the same if impulses are conducted, and the QRS complex may be usually widened. The P:QRS ratio varies 2:1, 3:1, and 4:1. Type II block is more dangerous than Type I because it may progress to complete AV block and may produce Stokes-Adams syncope. Individuals with a Type II block often need physical therapy, as they may have congestive heart failure or other symptoms.

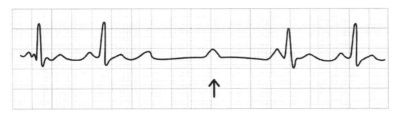

35

- **Third-degree AV block** is a complete heart block characterized on an ECG as more P waves than QRS complexes, with no clear relationship between them. The atrial rate is 2-3 times the pulse rate, so the PR interval is irregular. This can occur subsequent to many types of cardiac disease, including anteroseptal MI and coronary artery disease, as well as other issues like conduction problems or electrolyte imbalance. These patients have severe CHF and need medical attention.

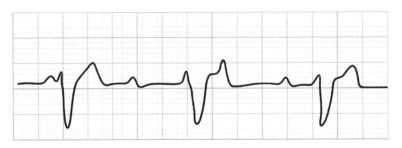

> **Review Video: AV Heart Blocks**
> Visit mometrix.com/academy and enter code: 487004

VALVULAR HEART DISEASE

There are three basic types of valvular heart disease:

- **Stenosis**: The narrowing of a valve.
- **Regurgitation**: Reverse blood flow through a valve due to incomplete closure.
- **Prolapse**: The displacement of a valve due to enlarged cusps.

The end result of valvular heart disease can be pumping problems or heart failure. Valvular heart disease usually occurs at the aortic valve or mitral valve. Aortic stenosis, chronic aortic regurgitation, and acute aortic regurgitation are common manifestations involving the aortic valve, all of which can be reasons for left ventricular failure and all of which can be indicated by murmurs. Stenosis, chronic regurgitation, acute regurgitation, and prolapse all often occur at the mitral valve. An enlarged left atrium suggests possible mitral stenosis or chronic regurgitation with pulmonary vascular congestion as a major symptom. Mitral valve prolapse usually presents as a systolic click, but symptoms may be absent or present simply as fatigue or palpitation.

MYOCARDIAL HEART DISEASE

Myocardial heart diseases, also known as cardiomyopathies, are disorders in which the heart muscle, or myocardium, is affected in some way. Functionally, there are three types of cardiomyopathies:

- The **dilated type**, in which the ventricle is dilated and contractility is diminished; results in systolic dysfunction.
- The **hypertrophic type**, in which the ventricular myocardium is thickened resulting in less compliance and filling; adversely affects diastolic function.
- The **restrictive type**, in which there is endocrinal scarring of the ventricles, decreases both compliance during diastole and contractile force during systole.

Cardiomyopathies are also often classified in terms of their etiology, for example, as inflammatory (infarctions due to viruses or bacteria), metabolic (often due to diabetes), genetic (such as Duchene's muscular dystrophy), infiltrative (due to malignancies or sarcoidosis), physical agents (such as radiation or hypothermia), and others.

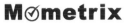

PERICARDIAL HEART DISEASE

Pericardial heart diseases are the result of some sort of issue with the pericardium, the fibrous sac enclosing the heart. The four basic types are acute pericarditis (inflammation of the pericardium), constrictive pericarditis, chronic pericardial effusion, and pericardial tamponade.

- Patients with **acute pericarditis** have pericardial friction rub, retrosternal chest pain, difficulty breathing, a cough, difficulty swallowing, fever, and chills.
- **Constrictive pericarditis** is suggested by jugular vein distention. Symptoms include abdominal swelling, peripheral edema, vague retrosternal chest pain, shortness of breath, dizziness, and pulmonary venous congestion.
- People with **chronic pericardial effusion (fluid)** have muffled heart sounds and possibly pericardial friction rub. They tend to have a vague fullness in their anterior chest, a cough, hoarseness, and difficulty swallowing.
- **Pericardial tamponade** occurs when the fluid buildup is enough to increase and equalize pressures to parts of the heart thus reducing cardiac output. Signs include jugular vein distention and cardiomegaly (heart enlargement). Patients present symptoms associated with low cardiac output, such as dyspnea, dizziness, and possibly retrosternal chest pain.

On an ECG, all of these diseases show a decreased QRS voltage.

HEART FAILURE

Heart failure is a decrease in cardiac output as reflected in a decreased ejection fraction. The heart cannot pump enough blood to meet bodily needs so that if left untreated, death can result. Heart failure is usually called congestive heart failure (CHF), which is descriptive of the buildup of blood in the heart that often enlarges it.

CHF can be classified as a left-sided heart failure, where the left ventricle is affected and there is back flow to the lungs, or right-sided, in which the right-side failure causes back flow to the systemic venous system. It can also be described as a high- or low-output failure, meaning that it is either secondary to renal system failure (i.e., fluid is not being sufficiently filtered off) or that the output is so low that circulation cannot be sustained. Heart failure can also be a systolic or diastolic dysfunction.

Many signs suggest CHF, including cold, pallid, possibly cyanotic extremities; peripheral edema; distention of the jugular vein; chest rales; an enlarged liver; and sinus tachycardia. The patient may have gained weight and have a diminished capacity for exercise and physical work. Many symptoms are breathing-related, including shortness of breath, spastic nighttime breathing, rapid breathing, orthopnea, and cough. The heart during inadequate circulation is said to be "decompensated" as opposed to "compensated" when medically stabilized.

AHA CLASSIFICATIONS OF HEART FAILURE

The American Heart Association (AHA) places patients with heart failure into one of four classes based on objective assessment and functional capacity. They are as follows:

- **Class I**: The patient is essentially asymptomatic during normal activities with no pulmonary congestion or peripheral hypotension. There is no restriction on activities, and prognosis is good.
- **Class II**: Symptoms appear with physical exertion but are usually absent at rest, resulting in some limitations of activities of daily living (ADLs). Slight pulmonary edema may be evident by basilar rales. Prognosis is good.

37

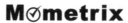

- **Class III**: Obvious limitations of ADLs and discomfort on any exertion. Prognosis is fair.
- **Class IV**: Symptoms at rest. Prognosis is poor.

DEKERLEGAND'S STAGING OF CONGESTIVE HEART FAILURE

Recently, staging for congestive heart failure was described by J. Dekerlegand (2007) as follows:

- **Stage A**: Patient is at risk for development of left ventricular dysfunction; treatment is directed toward modifying risk factors.
- **Stage B**: Patient has asymptomatic left ventricular dysfunction; management is focused on risk factor modification to avoid symptoms.
- **Stage C**: Patient presents with symptomatic left ventricular dysfunction; treatment is focused on mitigation of symptoms and thwarting disease progression.
- **Stage D**: Patient is diagnosed with advanced refractory disease; the condition is managed aggressively with drugs, surgical devices, and/or transplantation.

> **Review Video: Congestive Heart Failure**
> Visit mometrix.com/academy and enter code: 924118

PHARMACOLOGIC AND NON-PHARMACOLOGIC MANAGEMENT

THROMBOLYTIC THERAPY

Thrombolytic therapy is the intravenous use of thrombolytic agents during an acute myocardial infarction (MI). The basis of this therapy is that most individuals experiencing a MI have coronary artery thrombosis or blood clots. The therapy should ideally be given within six hours (risks may outweigh benefits if after 12 hours), unless the patient is at risk for excessive bleeding. The therapeutic agents administered fall into two classes. Fibrin-selective agents like tenecteplase and reteplase are preferred over non-selective ones like streptokinase due to the decrease in risk and ease of use.

PERCUTANEOUS TRANSLUMINAL CORONARY ANGIOPLASTY (PTCA)

Percutaneous transluminal coronary angioplasty (PTCA) is a procedure done to reperfuse coronary arteries blocked by plaque or an embolus. Cardiac catheterization is done with a hollow catheter (sheath), usually inserted into the femoral vein or artery, and fed through the vessels to the coronary arteries. When the atheroma is verified by fluoroscopy, a balloon-tipped catheter is fed over the sheath and the balloon is inflated with a contrast agent to a specified pressure to compress the atheroma. The balloon may be inflated a number of times to ensure that residual stenosis is <20%. Laser angioplasty using the excimer laser is also used to vaporize plaque. **Stents** may be inserted during the angioplasty to maintain patency. Stents may be flexible plastic or wire mesh and are typically placed over the catheter, which is inflated to expand the stent against the arterial wall. All patients with a stent must be discharged on aspirin, an antiplatelet, and a statin.

CORONARY ARTERY BYPASS GRAFTS AND TRANSMYOCARDIAL REVASCULARIZATION

Coronary artery bypass grafts and transmyocardial revascularization are two methods of revascularization of the myocardium in patients with cardiac disease. A coronary artery bypass graft (CABG) is indicated when there is complete blockage of the coronary artery or if percutaneous revascularization procedures are ineffective. The incisions are either minimally invasive or performed through a median sternotomy, and the blood vessels commonly used for the vascular graft are the saphenous vein or the left internal mammary artery (LIMA). Patients who have had a CABG with median sternotomy should keep upper-extremity use to a minimum for about two months afterwards.

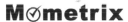

The other technique, transmyocardial laser revascularization, is indicated for patients who cannot endure CABG or angioplasty. It employs a catheter with a laser tip to construct channels from unblocked coronary arteries into a region of the myocardium where there is blockage. This treatment has proven effective in treating angina pain that isn't responsive to medications or in conjunction with minimally invasive CABG.

SECONDARY PROCEDURES FOLLOWING MYOCARDIAL REVASCULARIZATION

The types of secondary procedures typically performed after myocardial revascularization include:

- **Ablation procedures**: The use of a catheter to reach and remove ectopic foci using low-power, high-frequency alternating currents, possibly in conjunction with surgical ablation (the latter most commonly used for atrial fibrillation).
- **Implantation of a cardiac pacemaker or automatic implantable cardiac defibrillator**: The implantation on the myocardium of a unipolar or bipolar electrode to generate an action potential that controls arrhythmias.
- **Valve replacement**: Replacement in patients with valvular disease of the defective valve with a mechanical (more durable and long-lasting but often thrombogenic) or biologic valve (from a cadaver or animal tissue); typically involves median sternotomy for access.
- **Cardiac transplantation**: A procedure generally performed only on patients with end-stage cardiac disease.
- **Cardiac medications**: The use of drugs that fall into a number of categories, such as antiarrhythmic agents, anticoagulants, antihypertensives, fibrinolytics, and others.

PACEMAKERS

Both cardiac pacemakers and automatic implantable cardiac defibrillators (AICDs) are used to manage arrhythmias. Pacemakers use unipolar or bipolar electrodes on the myocardium to generate an action potential. They are utilized in patients with sinus node disorders, atrioventricular disorders, tachyarrhythmias, or when improved atrioventricular and/or biventricular synchrony is needed. Pacemakers are classified according to whether or not certain chambers are paced, sensed and triggered, or inhibited if sensed; whether or not there is rate modulation; and the location of multisite pacing. Rate modulation, the capacity to modulate heart rate based on activity levels or physiologic needs, is an important concept for physical therapists and their assistants. If there is no rate modulation, only low-level activity with small incremental changes should be performed; if there is rate modulation, then blood pressure must be watched when the patient's heart rate is near the upper limit of rate modulation.

An AICD is indicated for management of critical, uncontrollable ventricular arrhythmias, such as tachycardia or fibrillation. AICDs work by discerning the heart rhythm and then defibrillating the myocardium to establish normal rhythm.

Cardiac Physical Therapy Interventions

MEASURING PATIENT TOLERANCE OF PHYSICAL THERAPY ACTIVITIES

There are several parameters that can be used to gauge a patient's tolerance for a particular activity level.

- **Heart rate (HR) monitoring** is one of the best indications as heart rate and work are linearly related. HR is used in a number of ways, such as choosing activities that result in a HR 20-30 bpm above resting or within a safe range (typically 60-80% of the maximum).

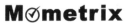

- **Heart rate recovery (HRR),** which is the difference in heart rate at its peak during activity and 60 seconds later, should normally be more than 18 bpm or 12 bpm depending on whether or not there has been a cool-down period.
- **Blood pressure (BP)** is also monitored to make sure it does not indicate extreme hypertension (>180 mmHg systolic, >110 mmHg diastolic) or that the systolic component does not go down more than 10 mmHg below resting. BP can also be used to determine intensity in patients with non-rate-modulated pacemakers.
- The **rate pressure product (RPP)** can be calculated as (HR × systolic BP) to provide an indication of myocardial oxygen demand.
- **Auscultation** can be used to listen for normal and abnormal heart sounds and breath sounds.
- **Continuous monitoring with an electrocardiogram** (ECG) is generally done during conditioning exercises like treadmill use for cardiac patients. The main reason an ECG is performed is to identify divergences from a patient's normal heart rhythm and potential decline in cardiac status. ECG indications of declining status include ST changes, increased occurrence or areas of premature ventricular contractions (PVCs), progression of heart blockage, and development of atrial fibrillation.

BORG SCALES FOR MEASURING PATIENT TOLERANCE

Borg scales are used to measure a **patient's rate of perceived exertion (RPE)** during exercises. There are three Borg Scales: the Borg RPE Scale, the Borg CR10 Scale, and the Borg CR100 Scale. The Borg RPE (rating of perceived exertion) Scale is the gold standard for subjective rating by the patient of exercise intensity, breathlessness, or muscle fatigue; it uses a scale from 6 to 20. The Borg CR10 and Borg CR100 (centiMax) Scales also measure RPE, just using different scales indicated by their names. Borg CR10 uses a scale of 1 to 10; Borg CR100 uses 1 to 100. These subjective measurements are useful because, in general, it is recommended that individuals only exercise to point 13 on the Borg RPE or point 5 on the Borg CR10 Scales. They are also very useful for patients taking beta-blockers because these individuals cannot be monitored via heart rate as these drugs regulate heart activity.

INDICATIONS OF PATIENT INSTABILITY

Regardless of whether an individual's underlying cardiac issue is related to ischemia, pump failure, or congestive heart failure, patients present with similar symptoms during activity or exercise if they are unstable. Unstable congestive heart or pump failure can present as a greater than 10 mmHg increase in pulmonary artery pressure and/or a deviation in central venous pressure of more than 6 mmHg. Otherwise, unstable patients can be observed to have cyanosis, sweating, nasal flaring, increased use of accessory muscles for respiration, a subjective increase in RPE, pallor, confusion, and symptoms of ischemia, notably angina (chest pain). Patients usually have symptoms of congestive heart failure whether or not that is the underlying problem. Certain ECG changes occur with instability, including ST segment changes, development of multifocal PVCs, and increased occurrence of ventricular ectopy. Instability is also indicated by a systolic BP drop of more than 10 mmHg, a diastolic BP change in either direction of more than 10 mmHg, and a heart rate drop of more than 10 bpm.

INTERVENTIONS

If a cardiac patient is unstable, they should receive medical attention before any physical therapy is performed. Indications that a patient is unstable and physical therapy should be withheld include the presence of decompensated congestive heart failure, heart blocks that are either third-degree or second-degree with premature ventricular contractions (PVCs), excessive or multifocal PVCs, a dissecting aortic aneurysm, recent onset atrial fibrillation, or chest pain with new ST segment

40

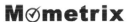

changes. In addition to these, there are other situations that suggest instability and modification or withholding of physical therapy. These include a resting heart rate of more than 100 bpm, a myocardial infarction or its extension within the last two days, ventricular ectopy or atrial fibrillation while resting, the presence of uncontrollable metabolic diseases, patient psychosis, or indications of resting hypertension or hypotension. These are defined as blood pressure readings of greater than 140 mmHg systolic/90 mmHg diastolic for hypertension and less than 80 mmHg systolic BP for hypotension.

OUTPATIENT CARDIAC REHABILITATION

BASIC ELEMENTS

Outpatient cardiac rehabilitation is geared toward helping patients manage cardiac disease, assisting patients with recovery after a myocardial infarction, or facilitating recovery after cardiovascular-related surgery. Patients can initiate outpatient cardiac rehab once they are medically stable and cleared to do so by a medical professional. Cardiac rehab will typically include exercise and education to help patients understand their condition, take steps to improve their health, and make lifestyle changes to facilitate a prolonged lifespan and improved quality of life. Programs usually involve a multidisciplinary healthcare team and include a medical evaluation, education about lifestyle factors that influence the condition, an exercise plan, and some form of ongoing support regarding mental health and coping strategies as needed. Providers also engage patients with discussions about plans for returning to work as applicable. Ideally, patients leave cardiac rehab with a strategy for maintaining a healthy lifestyle and reducing the risk of cardiovascular complications over the long term.

GOALS

Outpatient cardiac rehabilitation aims to develop an exercise program to improve cardiovascular fitness and strength, educate patients about lifestyle modifications that influence their condition, improve a patient's functional capacity for activities of daily living, develop stress management strategies, and make plans to return to work as applicable. Improving cardiovascular fitness and strength enables individuals to have the capacity to safely perform activities of daily living and work tasks, while also reducing risks for the occurrence or recurrence of cardiovascular emergencies. Educating patients about lifestyle factors such as nutrition, sleep hygiene, and smoking cessation also helps manage conditions and reduce the risk of future cardiac issues. Stress management strategies facilitate a means by which patients are able to manage their mental health while dealing with potentially long-term limitations of their condition. Healthcare providers can assist patients and employers with plans to return to work with modifications as necessary. Medical evaluations are utilized throughout the process to document progress toward these goals and make adjustments to the plan of care when required.

EXERCISES

Exercise programs within an outpatient cardiac rehabilitation program incorporate aerobic activity, strength training, and stretching. Aerobic exercise commonly includes walking, jogging, riding a bicycle, or rowing. The goal of aerobic exercises are to improve cardiorespiratory function and impart psychological benefits. Strength training usually focuses on upper and lower body strength and may include the use of bands, ankle weights, dumbbells, barbells, or weight machines. Examples of upper body strength exercises include overhead press, lateral raises, front raises, and rows. Examples of lower body strength exercises include sit-to-stands, marching, knee extensions, hamstring curls, and box lifts. Stretching exercises aim to improve range of motion to allow patients to more easily attain positions required for daily activities. Vital signs such as blood pressure and heart rate as well as rating of perceived exertion are objective and subjective metrics that are used during sessions to monitor the patient's response to exercise programming.

41

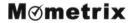

Vascular Physical Therapy Data Collection

PATIENT HISTORY

A physical examination that includes information relevant to the vascular system should incorporate specific components of history, inspection, palpation, auscultation, vascular tests, and diagnostic studies. The history should reveal pertinent medical history (for example, history of diabetes, hypertension, high lipid levels, etc.), exercise habits, use of tobacco or alcohol, and periods of lengthy bed rest or vascular surgery. A large part should be devoted to the documentation of pain because it can be indicative of vascular occlusion and claudication (reduced blood supply to the leg muscles). Therefore, pain in the extremities, nocturnal pain, pain at rest (suggesting advanced occlusion), intermittent claudication, and claudication in the buttock, hip, or thigh (a sign of obstruction in the aorta and iliac arteries) should all be detailed. The patient's history or current presence of edema, which also suggests vascular problems, should be documented.

VASCULAR DATA COLLECTION

During a vascular evaluation, the clinician should inspect certain features to determine the location and magnitude of vascular disease and whether it is localized in the arteries or veins. The clinician should observe the patient's extremities (particularly the legs) for discolorations in skin color at the distal extremities and nail beds, dilated or purplish veins, digital clubbing, patchy hair distribution, and the presence of cellulitis, petechiae spots, and/or skin lesions. Clinicians should also observe the patient for gait abnormalities, and edema or atrophy in extremities, in particular, should be carefully observed and documented. Bilateral peripheral edema suggests right-sided congestive heart failure; unilateral peripheral edema suggests chronic venous insufficiency, obstruction of lymphatics, or trauma. The physical therapist should use a tape measure to quantify the circumference of the person's forefoot, the smallest part above the ankle, the biggest part of the calf, and the mid-thigh with knee extended. Edema is implied if the metric differs more than 1 cm from a normal value or the measurement from the other side above the ankle or 2 cm at the calf.

PALPATION AND AUSCULTATION

The most important part of palpation for vascular function is measuring the peripheral pulses in terms of strength and rate. The typical peripheral pulses to evaluate are the carotid, brachial, radial, temporal, ulnar, femoral, popliteal, posterior tibial, and dorsalis pedis. Note that carotid arteries should not be palpated at the same time as that can reduce blood flow to the brain. Each pulse should be graded from 0 to +4. Weak peripheral pulses suggest decreased fluid volumes and possible corresponding upticks in heart and respiratory rates. Doppler may be indicated if pulses are not palpable to ensure perfusion to the extremity. However, some adults may have absent peripheral pulses. Patients with diabetes, hypertension, or peripheral vascular disease should have their pulses tested before, during, and after activity to look at changes. Palpation can also inform the physical therapist about pain at a particular site, the presence/absence of edema, the temperature of the skin, etc.

Auscultation for vascular function should include a measurement of systemic blood pressure and listening for bruits, the whooshing sounds associated with turbulent blood flow due to obstruction.

HEMATOLOGIC EVALUATION

A hematologic evaluation should include appropriate history, inspection, and palpation, as well as a number of laboratory studies. The history portion should address patient or familial history of anemia and other blood disorders, malignancies, hemorrhage, and infections. It should document presenting symptoms and their onset and should include questions regarding prior blood transfusions, chemotherapy, radiation therapy, drug therapy, environmental contact with toxins,

42

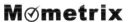

ease of bruising and wound healing, presence of night sweats or fever, and excessive bleeding or menstrual periods. The patient should be observed for general indications of malaise, presence of petechiae spots or ecchymosis (bruising), respiratory rate, and the color (pale or flushed) of the skin, mucous membranes, nail beds, and palm creases. The physician usually does the palpation portion of the examination, but the physical therapist might use palpation to evaluate bone and joint pain, range of motion, paresthesia, blood pressure, and heart rate, all of which could have some relevance to hematologic or vascular function. This information is then shared with the physical therapist assistant.

PERIPHERAL BLOOD SMEARS AND D-DIMER ASSAY

Peripheral blood smears are also taken to evaluate for hematologic abnormalities that may contribute to various vascular issues, and the three types of blood cells—red blood cells (RBCs), white blood cells (WBCs), and platelets—are observed microscopically. The parameters of interest are the size, shape, and hemoglobin distribution of RBCs, the percentage of immature cells among WBCs, and the number and shape of platelets.

The D-dimer assay is used to confirm disseminated intravascular coagulation (DIC) and deep vein thrombosis (DVT) as it is elevated in these conditions, as well as other conditions associated with thrombosis. The assay quantifies D-dimer, a fibrin degradation product that is correlated to blood clot formation.

DIAGNOSTIC TESTS FOR PERFUSION

Perfusion can be evaluated with three tests:

- **Capillary refill**: Grasp the toenail bed between the thumb and index finger and apply pressure for several seconds to cause blanching. Release the nail and count the seconds until the nail regains normal color. Arterial occlusion is indicated with times of more than 2-3 seconds. Check both feet and more than one nail bed.
- **Elevation pallor**: To assess arterial perfusion, this exam involves elevating the limb 30-40° for 15-60 seconds and monitoring whether color changes are observed. Pallor or gray color changes indicate occlusive disease. The condition is considered severe if color changes at 25 seconds, moderate if it occurs at 25-40 seconds, and mild at 40-60 seconds.
- **Ankle-Brachial Index (ABI)**: Calculation of the ratio between perfusion pressures in the lower leg and upper extremity helps check for evidence of arterial insufficiency. The patient lays down while blood pressure readings are taken in two spots for brachial readings (one on each arm) and two on the lower leg (dorsalis pedis and posterior tibial). The higher readings for each are used to calculate ABI as:
  - ABI = highest ankle pressure/highest brachial pressure
  - ABI ranges and their indications are:
    - ❖ >1.4: Abnormally high, may indicate calcification of vessel wall
    - ❖ 1.0–1.4: Normal reading, asymptomatic
    - ❖ 0.9–1.0: Low reading, but acceptable unless there are other indications of PAD
    - ❖ 0.8–0.9: Likely some arterial disease is present
    - ❖ 0.5–0.8: Moderate arterial disease
    - ❖ < 0.5: Severe arterial disease

BRODIE-TRENDELENBURG TEST

The Brodie-Trendelenburg test for vascular function, also known as the retrograde filling test, is used to look at whether varicosities are due to superficial or deep veins and their valves. The distended veins in question are marked while the patient is standing. The person then lies down and raises the leg for approximately a minute to drain the veins. The patient stands up again, and the physical therapist observes the time it takes to fill up the veins. Veins should normally take a minimum of 30 seconds to refill. If they fill more quickly, the patient should lie down again, elevating the leg for a minute. A tourniquet is put on the upper thigh while the patient is lying, then the patient stands, the tourniquet is taken off, and vein filling is observed again. Rapid filling at less than 30 seconds suggests the perforating vein and deep vein valves are incompetent. In order to locate the site of the incompetent valve, the procedure involving the tourniquet is repeated below the knee and around the upper calf. If rapid filling (< 30 seconds) persists, superficial vein valves allowing backflow should be presumed.

MANUAL COMPRESSION TEST, ALLEN'S TEST, AND HOMAN'S SIGN

Additional vascular tests include:

- **Manual compression test**: Used to distinguish whether a valve in a vein is competent or not, this test involves palpation of the dilated vein and compression and palpation with the other hand about 8 inches higher. The absence of impulse is normal, while the presence of impulse at the higher spot indicates incompetent valves in the segment.
- **Allen's test**: To evaluate the patency of arteries (radial and ulnar) and circulation in the hand, the patient is asked to bend their arm, holding the hand above the elbow. The clinician compresses the radial and ulnar arteries at the wrist, while the patient clenches the fist then opens it, and one of the arteries is released (repeated later with the other artery). The released artery area should change from blanched to flushed in a matter of seconds if circulation is normal (positive); if abnormal, local circulation is deficient (negative).
- **Homan's sign**: For the detection of deep vein thrombosis, the calf muscle is squeezed or the foot is rapidly bent back. If the patient experiences pain, deep vein thrombosis is suggested. There is a high degree of false positives with this test.

NONINVASIVE DIAGNOSTIC TESTS

There are both noninvasive and invasive studies that can be performed to diagnose vascular abnormalities. The noninvasive vascular diagnostic studies for the evaluation of vascular flow include:

- **Exercise testing**: Measurement of ankle pressure and peripheral vascular resistance after exercise; lowered ankle pressure is suggestive of arterial disease.
- **Doppler ultrasound**: Local skin application with a probe of high-frequency, low-intensity sound waves; used to detect, determine the direction of, and characterize blood flow.
- **Color duplex scanning or imaging**: Use of ultrasound with a pulsed Doppler detector; visualizes vessels and possible plaques; generates distinctive color changes in regions.
- **Plethysmography**: Measures volumetric changes, in this case, the volume of blood distal to a particular area to indicate occlusion.
- **Computed tomography (CT)**: X-ray imaging technique used, in this case, to visualize the arterial wall.
- **Magnetic resonance imaging (MRI)**: Imaging technique using electromagnetic radiation to visualize soft tissues, in this instance, the arterial system.
- **Magnetic resonance angiography (MRA)**: Utilization of blood as a contrast medium, along with magnetic resonance imaging, to look at the structure of and blood flow through major blood vessels.

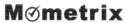

INVASIVE DIAGNOSTIC TESTS

Contrast angiography or arteriography is the only frequently used type of invasive vascular diagnostic study. It involves injection of a radiopaque dye into the brachial, axillary, femoral, or lumbar arteries; the acquisition of a radiograph; and then, often, use of digital subtraction angiography to remove bony structures from the image. Contrast angiography is useful for the visualization of blood flow dynamics, vascular anatomy, and tumors. It is usually done prior to or during interventions like angioplasty, surgical bypasses, or thrombolytic therapy. Possible complications may be associated with the injected contrast agent (such as anaphylactic sensitivity reactions), the puncture site (for example, local thrombosis), or the catheter used (these must be checked). Patients who have undergone this procedure should rest for four to eight hours. During this time, they should be given IV fluids to get rid of the contrast dye and monitored for BUN, creatinine, and vital signs. Pressure dressings should be applied at the injection site (observing for hematomas). Patients previously on heparin should not be restarted on the medication until a minimum of four hours after the procedure.

Vascular Diseases/Conditions that Impact Effective Treatment

ARTERIAL VS. VENOUS VASCULAR DISORDERS

Characteristics of peripheral arterial and venous insufficiency are listed below:

- Arterial insufficiency
  - **Pain**: Ranging from intermittent claudication to severe and constant shooting pain
  - **Pulses**: Weak or absent
  - **Skin**: Rubor on dependency, but pallor of foot on elevation; pale, shiny, and cool skin with loss of hair on toes and foot; nails thick and ridged
  - **Ulcers**: Painful, deep, circular, often necrotic ulcers on toe tips, toe webs, heels, or other pressure areas
  - **Edema**: Minimal
- Venous insufficiency
  - **Pain**: Aching/cramping
  - **Pulses**: Strong/present
  - **Skin**: Brownish discoloration around ankles and anterior tibial area
  - **Ulcers**: Varying degrees of pain in superficial, irregular ulcers on medial or lateral malleolus and sometimes the anterior tibial area
  - **Edema**: Moderate to severe

ATHEROSCLEROSIS

Atherosclerosis is an arterial disorder in which blood flow is impeded by the progressive narrowing of blood vessels due to hemorrhaging, cellular proliferation, and the deposition of lipid-containing plaques. There are a number of risk factors predisposing individuals to atherosclerosis, including hypertension, diabetes, high cholesterol, obesity, cigarette use, family history, and male gender. Predictors include C-reactive protein (CRP), waist circumference, and weight gain. The vessel stenosis causes blood flow turbulence and diminished perfusion distal to it. The major symptom, pain, is generally not observed until the blood flow is reduced by at least 50%. Other signs include reduced or missing peripheral pulses, existence of bruits upon auscultation of larger arteries, cool and pale skin, high blood pressure, and pain in the toes at rest and in the calf or leg when walking (known as intermittent claudicating). Treatment modalities may incorporate risk factor changes, use of anticoagulant and thrombolytic drugs, surgical resection, and grafting. Atherosclerosis in the extremities may be referred to as peripheral vascular or arterial disease (PVD, PAD).

INTERMITTENT CLAUDICATION AND PSEUDOCLAUDICATION

Intermittent claudication refers to tight, cramping pain in the extremities, generally the calves, due to an inadequate blood supply to the muscles. The condition is caused by atherosclerosis or narrowing of the blood vessels. It is induced by exercise and alleviated by rest, standing still, or stopping the activity. The location of the pain experienced is found on one side only, in the buttock, hip, thigh, calf, and/or foot. Intermittent claudicating almost always occurs at a predictable interval when walking on the level, which may or may not decrease when walking uphill or increase when walking downhill.

Pseudoclaudication is pain that is neurologic in derivation, such as stenosis of the lumbar canal or disc disease. Associated leg pain is bilateral, and there is often back pain. People with pseudoclaudication feel pain when standing, which is alleviated by sitting and may or may not be induced by activity. It is often mistaken for intermittent claudication as the pain may be similar in nature; or, instead, the pain may be characterized by tingling, weakness, and clumsiness. The onset of pseudoclaudication is unpredictable and, contrary to the intermittent type, occurs later when walking uphill and earlier when walking downhill.

ANEURYSM

Abdominal aortic aneurysms (AAA) are usually related to atherosclerosis, but may also result from Marfan syndrome, Ehlers-Danlos disease, and connective tissue disorders. Rupture usually does not allow time for emergent repair, so identifying and correcting before rupture is essential. Different classification systems are used to describe the type and degree of dissection. Common classification:

- **DeBakey classification** uses anatomic location as the focal point:
  - Type I begins in the ascending aorta but may spread to include the aortic arch and the descending aorta (60%). This is also considered a proximal lesion or Stanford type A.
  - Type II is restricted to the ascending aorta (10-15%). This is also considered a proximal lesion or Stanford type A.
  - Type III is restricted to the descending aorta (25-30%). This is considered a distal lesion or Stanford type B.
- Types I and II are thoracic, and type III is abdominal.

AORTIC DISSECTION

A **dissecting aortic aneurysm** occurs when the wall of the aorta is torn and blood flows between the layers of the wall, dilating and weakening it until it risks rupture (which has a 90% mortality). Aortic aneurysms are more than twice as common in males as females, but females have a higher mortality rate, possibly due to increased age at diagnosis.

Patients with aortic dissection can present with acute, excruciating pain in the chest or upper back, which moves toward the path of dissection; fainting, diminished, or absent pulses; a murmur associated with aortic regurgitation; and neurological issues. Diagnosis is made by transesophageal echocardiography (TEE) or CT scanning as electrocardiograms readings are very vague. Aneurysms are currently managed via surgical resection, graft replacement, or endovascular repair.

ARTERIAL THROMBOSIS AND ARTERIAL EMBOLI

Arterial thrombosis is the adhesion and aggregation of platelets resulting in clotting in arterial regions of low or stagnant blood flow. An embolus is a mass, generally a blood clot, which blocks a blood vessel. When a thrombosis breaks free from its vessel into circulation it is referred to as an embolus. Sometimes these emboli can lodge in the heart and result stagnant or erratic blood flow.

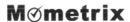

About 80% of emboli are cardiac in origin, due mostly to atrial fibrillation or myocardial infarction. Some combination of thrombi and/or emboli is the result. Treatment regimens include anticoagulation measures, with or without partial surgical removal of the atherosclerotic regions, or use of antithrombotic agents (such as tissue factors), possibly in conjunction with aspirin, thienopyridine, and/or warfarin. Patients experiencing an acute arterial embolus must be treated immediately.

HYPERTENSION

Hypertension is the elevation of both components of arterial blood pressure while resting. Hypertension can be secondary to a disease process, or essential (unrelated to an explicit medical cause). Some predisposing factors are genetics, smoking, obesity, diabetes, atherosclerosis, a high-fat or high-sodium diet, and vasomediator imbalance. Causes of secondary hypertension are usually related to hereditary coarctation (constriction) of the aorta, the pituitary disorder Cushing's disease, renovascular diseases, and adrenal tumors. Hypertension can affect the brain, causing cerebrovascular accidents or encephalopathy; the eyes, manifesting as blurred or impaired vision or encephalopathy; the kidneys, in the form of renal insufficiency, possibly progressing to renal failure; and the heart, as myocardial infarction, congestive heart failure, myocardial hypertrophy, or dysrhythmias. Management tools include behavioral modification, exercise, and drugs, such as diuretics, beta and calcium-channel blockers, vasodilators, and angiogenesis-converting enzyme inhibitors.

SYSTEMIC VASCULITIS, RAYNAUD'S DISEASE, AND RAYNAUD'S PHENOMENON

Systemic vasculitis refers to tissue damage and the eventual narrowing of blood vessels due to inflammation. The underlying causes of systemic vasculitis are often related to the immune system, as well as infectious agents, tumors, drugs, or unknown causes. Vasculitis can secondarily result in thrombosis, aneurysm development, hemorrhage, occlusion, weight loss, and/or generalized malaise.

Raynaud's disease and **phenomenon** both occur in a cold environment, the former with idiopathic or unknown origin and the latter due to autoimmune, myeloproliferative, or arterial occlusive disorders. The characteristic sign of both is a color change in the digits or tip of the nose from white to blue to red (corresponding to vasoconstriction, cyanosis, and vasodilation). These changes occur symmetrically in Raynaud's disease and erratically in Raynaud's phenomenon. Raynaud's disease is not serious and is often controllable, but Raynaud's phenomenon can lead to atrophy of fat pads and, eventually, gangrene. Management includes a conservative means of warming and shielding affected areas, exercise, administration of calcium-channel blockers and sympatholytics, alternative medical procedures, and diets plentiful in antioxidants and fish oils.

ADDITIONAL TYPES OF SYSTEMIC VASCULITIS

The known types of systemic vasculitis in addition to Raynaud's disease and phenomenon are:

- **Polyarteritis nodosa**: Acute necrotizing vasculitis of small or medium arteries; possibly due to hepatitis B virus infection. Characteristic manifestations include skin lesions, vasculitic neuropathy, and aneurysm development. This is managed with corticosteroids, cytotoxic, and antiviral drugs
- **Warner's granulomatosis**: Granulomatous destruction of small and medium blood vessels, particularly in the respiratory tract and kidneys. Symptoms are similar to pneumonia. This is treated with immunosuppressive drugs, corticosteroids, and, if needed, anti-infective agents

- **Giant cell arteritis (GCA)**: Granulomatous destruction of internal elastic lamina of larger arteries. The cause is unknown. GCA commonly presents as temporal arthritis characterized by headache, visual disturbances, jaw and tongue soreness, and possibly polymyalgia rheumatica. It can also manifest as Takayasu's arteritis, mainly in upper extremities.
- **Thromboangiitis obliterans (Buerger's disease)**: Thrombotic, abscessed occlusions of small and medium arteries of distal extremities, usually resulting from collagen or autoimmune disorder. It is associated with heavy cigarette use. Symptoms include rest pain and intermittent claudication in feet. Buerger's disease is treated with smoking cessation, corticosteroids, vasodilators, anticoagulants, etc.

Complex Regional Pain Syndrome

Complex regional pain syndrome (CRPS) is an uncommon disorder of the extremities that can occur after healing post-trauma or surgery. Undiminished sensory nerve signals to the spinal cord cause augmented sympathetic signals to the extremities. CRPS usually occurs in three stages:

- **Stage 1, the acute phase**: Characterized by pain, swelling, and temperature changes from warm to cold.
- **Stage 2, the dystrophic phase**: Where the pain broadens out and there is progressive degeneration of tissue resulting in possible muscle wasting, osteoporosis, lessened range of motion, etc.
- **Stage 3, the atrophic or chronic phase**: Characterized by atrophy, functional impairment, and permanent damage.

CRPS is managed with physical and/or occupational therapy, pharmacologic or surgical interventions to block the sympathetic nerve system, electrical stimulation of the spinal cord, vitamin C, and drugs like baclofen and bisphosphonates.

Compartment Syndrome

Compartment syndrome occurs when there is an increase in the amount of pressure within a grouping of muscles, nerves, and blood vessels resulting in compromised blood flow to muscles and nerves. This is a medical emergency. If left untreated, tissue ischemia and eventual tissue death will occur. Compartment syndrome most often occurs after a fracture, particularly a long bone fracture, but can also occur with crushing syndrome and rhabdomyolysis. Risk factors include lower extremity trauma, massive tissue injury, venous obstruction, the use of certain medications (anticoagulants), burns and compressive dressings or casts. Compartment syndrome can affect the hand, forearm, upper arm, abdomen, and lower extremities. It can be acute or chronic in nature with acute compartment syndrome requiring immediate intervention.

Signs and symptoms: Intense pain, decreased sensation and paresthesia, firmness at the affected site, swelling and tightness at the affected site, pallor and pulselessness (late signs).

Diagnosis: Physical assessment and the measurement of intra-compartmental pressures.

Management: The goal of treatment in compartment syndrome is decompression and the restoration of perfusion to the affected area. Surgical fasciotomy is often indicated to relieve pressure and prevent tissue death. Fasciotomy involves the opening of the skin and muscle fascia to release the pressure within the compartment and restore blood flow to the area.

Prevention: Leave large abdominal wounds open to drain, delay casting on affected extremities, and use flexible casts. Watch circumferential burns closely and perform frequent neurovascular checks on those at risk.

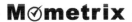

VARICOSE VEINS

Varicose veins, a venous disorder, are characterized by persistent dilation of veins. They are initially caused by the deterioration of the venous walls, which is followed by inadequate closure of valve cusps. There are two types: **primary varicose veins**, which stem from the superficial veins, and **secondary varicose veins**, which arise in the deep and perforating veins. People are at risk for primary varicose veins if they are female, have familial history of them, have had phlebitis (inflammation of the vein), or are in situations that prolong venous stasis, like pregnancy or occupations requiring prolonged standing. Primary varicose veins are generally bilateral, while secondary varicose veins are typically unilateral. Varicose veins are usually visible externally and may bleed profusely if traumatized. Varicose veins can be treated surgically by ligation and stripping, sclerotherapy, behavioral changes, weight loss, elevation of the feet several times daily, use of support stockings, measured exercise, and/or performance of bathing rituals at night.

VENOUS THROMBOSIS AND PULMONARY EMBOLISM

In venous thrombosis, blood clots form in the superficial or deep veins (DVT), potentially developing into a pulmonary embolism (PE). DVT is a consequence of venous stasis, damage to the vein's endothelium, and/or hypercoagulability. Risk factors include interventions (surgery, central venous catheters, etc.), cardiac issues (hypertension, varicose veins, heart failure, etc.), obesity, and others. A patient presenting with local pain and swelling, dilated veins, redness, warmth, tightness, and minimal fever should be suspected of DVT. DVT is usually diagnosed with ultrasound, although the most specific and sensitive method is magnetic resonance imaging. A positive Homan's sign, in combination with local swelling, redness, and warmth, is fairly diagnostic for DVT. DVT is initially treated with the anticoagulant heparin or, if contraindicated, an inferior vena cava (IVC) filter placed between the thrombus and the lungs to prevent PE. Other treatments include thrombolytic drugs (streptokinase, urokinase) and surgical thrombectomy. PE, blockage of a pulmonary artery or capillary, can lead to V/Q mismatch, decreased oxygen pressure and oxyhemoglobin saturation, hypoxemia, and, ultimately, pulmonary hypertension or right congestive heart failure. Physical therapy should not be done without medical clearance for DVT and discontinued if a PE develops.

CHRONIC VENOUS INSUFFICIENCY AND POSTPHLEBITIC SYNDROME

Chronic venous insufficiency and postphlebitic syndrome are two venous disorders with analogous causes and signs. The origin of each is valvular dysfunction resulting from venous thrombosis destruction and, to a lesser extent, obstruction of the venous outflow. About half of patients with deep venous thrombosis (DVT) develop one of these disorders within five years. Both are characterized by chronic swollen limbs, ulcerations due to venous stasis, and skin changes. These changes often include hemosiderosis, in which the skin develops a gray-brown hyperpigmentation due to the disintegration of extravasated red blood cells, and/or lipodermatosis, fibrosis or toughening of soft tissues in the lower extremities. Management strategies include elevation of the lower extremities above heart level several times daily for 10-15 minutes, the use of compression dressings or stockings, avoidance of pressure sources above the legs, skin hygiene and ulceration care, exercises that assist muscles with pumping venous blood, and surgical ligation of veins.

ANEMIA

Anemia is an erythrocytic disorder in which the numbers of red blood cells (RBCs) are depressed relative to normal due to diminished production, abnormal maturation, or augmented destruction. Types caused by decreased RBC production, increased destruction, or blood loss include:

- **Aplastic anemia**: This condition is characterized by diminished RBC production (also WBCs and platelets) subsequent to bone marrow damage. RBCs are normal or macrocytic (large). Possible signs include fatigue, dyspnea, evidence of bleeding (petechiae, fecal blood, heavy menses, gums, etc.), pallor, fever, and/or sore throat. Management includes transfusion, bone marrow transplantation, corticosteroids, antibiotics, etc.
- **Hemolytic anemia**: Patients with this disorder undergo the destruction or premature removal of RBCs; the hemolysis can occur intravascularly or extravascularly. Hemolytic anemia may be caused by a genetic defect related to the RBC structure or membrane or can be autoimmune in nature. Signs include fatigue, nausea, fever, chills, low urine output, jaundice, pain in the abdomen or back, and splenomegaly. The condition is managed with fluids, transfusion, corticosteroids, appendectomy, and elimination of the causative factor.

POSTHEMORRHAGIC ANEMIA AND ANEMIA OF CHRONIC DISEASE

Red blood cells (RBCs) are depleted (and sometimes abnormal) in anemia. Posthemorrhagic anemia is caused by rapid blood loss from some type of trauma. The symptoms depend on the percentage of blood loss. A 20-30% loss presents as faintness, hypotension, and rapid heart rate upon exertion. A person with 30-40% blood loss will have additional symptoms, such as dyspnea, clamminess, low urine output, and possibly unconsciousness. When blood loss reaches 40-50%, shock and possibly death can occur. Patients with posthemorrhagic anemia are managed with IV and oral fluids, transfusions, bleeding control, and supplemental oxygen.

About half of hospitalized patients and many individuals with inflammatory or neoplastic disorders or chronic infections have anemia of chronic disease (ACD). ACD usually requires no treatment.

IRON DEFICIENCY ANEMIA

Iron deficiency anemia is an extremely common type of anemia caused by abnormal red blood cell maturation. Other types associated with abnormal maturation include vitamin B_{12} anemia, folic acid anemia, and sickle cell anemia. Iron deficiency anemia occurs when iron storage in the bone marrow is decreased through another cause. The reduction encourages production of abnormal RBCs that are microcytic (small) and microchromic (less colored). Some of the initial causes include blood loss (including menses), pregnancy, a diet deficient in iron, and diminished iron absorption in the gastrointestinal tract. Iron-deficiency anemia can present as fatigue, headache, faintness, difficulty swallowing, softening of the nails, strange cravings, and/or pallid palms, earlobes, or conjunctivae. Management includes identification of the source, iron supplementation, and nutritional advice.

VITAMIN B$_{12}$ AND FOLIC ACID ANEMIA

Vitamin B$_{12}$ and folic acid anemias are two types of anemia that result with decreased levels of nutrients. Both cause production of RBCs that are normal in color but macrocytic (large).

- **Vitamin B$_{12}$ anemia** is caused by poor absorption of that vitamin due to enteritis, iliac disease, Crohn's disease, pancreatic insufficiency, or an associated type of anemia called pernicious anemia in which there is no intrinsic factor to bind vitamin B$_{12}$. Patients often have icterus, a yellow discoloration in certain areas due to increased blood bilirubin, as well as diarrhea, anorexia, oral ulcers, and/or neurologic changes. Diagnosis includes clinical findings, diminished serum vitamin B$_{12}$ levels, high lactate dehydrogenase and mean corpuscular volume (MCV), and a positive urine Schilling test. This anemia is treated with B$_{12}$ supplementation and nutritional advice.
- **Folic acid or folate deficiency**, due to insufficient intake, presents very similarly to vitamin B$_{12}$ deficiency minus the neurologic issues. It is identified by clinical findings, low serum folate levels, and high lactate dehydrogenase and MCV. Patients are given folic acid supplements.

SICKLE CELL ANEMIA

Sickle cell disease is a recessive genetic disorder of chromosome 11, causing hemoglobin to be defective so that red blood cells (RBCs) are sickle-shaped and inflexible, resulting in their accumulating in small vessels and causing painful blockage. While normal RBCs survive 120 days, sickled cells may survive only 10-20 days, stressing the bone marrow that cannot produce fast enough and resulting in severe anemia. There are 5 variations of sickle cell disease, with sickle cell anemia the most severe. Different types of crises occur (aplastic, hemolytic, vaso-occlusive, and sequestrating), which can cause infarctions in organs, severe pain, damage to organs, and rapid enlargement of liver and spleen. Complications include anemia, acute chest syndrome, congestive heart failure, strokes, delayed growth, infections, pulmonary hypertension, liver and kidney disorders, retinopathy, seizures, and osteonecrosis. Sickle cell disease occurs almost exclusively in African Americans in the United States, with 8-10% carriers.

> **Review Video: Sickle Cell Disease**
> Visit mometrix.com/academy and enter code: 603869

If physical therapy is performed, oximetry is suggested to measure oxygenation and exercise intensity.

POLYCYTHEMIA

Polycythemia vera is a condition in which there is abnormal production of blood cells in the bone marrow. Erythrocytes (red blood cells) are primarily affected. The disease is more common in men older than 40 years. Polycythemia may be primary or secondary, related to conditions causing hypoxia. The blood increases in viscosity, resulting in a number of **symptoms**:

- Dizziness, headache, weakness, and fatigue
- Dyspnea, especially when supine
- Flushing of skin, blue-tinged skin discoloration, and red lesions
- Itching after warm bath
- Left upper abdominal fullness and splenomegaly
- Phlebitis from blood clots
- Vision disturbances
- Complications include stroke, hemorrhage, and heart failure

51

Diagnosis includes CBC with differential, chemistry panel, bone marrow biopsy, and Vitamin B_{12} level. Red cell mass will be more than 25% above normal.

Management includes:

- **Phlebotomy** to remove 500 mL (lesser amounts for children) of blood to decrease blood viscosity, repeated weekly until hematocrit stable (less than 45%)
- Referral for **chemotherapy** (hydroxyurea) to suppress marrow production
- **Interferon** to decrease need for phlebotomy

NEUTROPENIA

Neutropenia is identified as a **polymorphonuclear neutrophil count** equal to or less than 500/mL. **Chronic neutropenia** is a sustained condition of minimal neutrophils lasting 3 or more months. Neutropenia may occur from a decreased production of **white blood cells** (e.g., from chemotherapy or radiation therapy). It may also occur from a loss of white blood cells from autoimmune disease processes. Neutropenia is silent but dangerous. It leaves essentially no neutrophils to fight any threat of infection. Neutrophils make up as much as 70% of the white blood cells circulating in the blood. Neutropenia can be the cause of a septic situation, which can be life-threatening. Up to 70% of patients experiencing a fever while in a neutropenic state will die within 48 hours if not treated aggressively.

DISSEMINATED INTRAVASCULAR COAGULATION (DIC)

Disseminated intravascular coagulation (DIC) is a potentially fatal thrombocytic syndrome characterized by both hemorrhaging and blood clot formation. It occurs most often after severe infections, in particular subsequent to gram-negative bacterial sepsis, as well as following some type of trauma or formation of antigen-antibody complexes. The process involved is multifaceted, starting with fibrin deposition (and excessive clotting) in the circulation and associated organ and RBC damage. This is followed by a number of events resulting from the subsequent depletion of clotting factors, namely platelet consumption and activation of clotting factors and plasmin, resulting in hemorrhage. Many symptoms that involve hemorrhage, thrombus formation, and/or organ failure in numerous bodily systems can suggest DIC. These systems include cardiopulmonary, renal, integumentary, gastrointestinal, and neurologic. Diagnosis includes presence of an elevated D-dimer, low platelet counts (thrombocytopenia), prolonged PT and APTT, and low fibrinogen levels. Patients with DIC are typically treated with fluid control, oxygen, transfusion (if there is ongoing bleeding), and measures to sustain hemodynamics and the cardiovascular system. Heparin therapy is sometimes used, but this is controversial.

HEMOPHILIA

Hemophilia is an inherited disorder in which the person lacks adequate clotting factors. There are three types:

- **Type A**: lack of clotting factor VIII (90% of cases)
- **Type B**: lack of clotting factor IX
- **Type C**: lack of clotting factor XI (affects both sexes, rarely occurs in the United States)

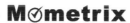

Both Type A and B are usually X-linked disorders, affecting only males. The severity of the disease depends on the amount of clotting factor in the blood.

Symptoms:

- Bleeding with severe trauma or stress (mild cases)
- Unexplained bruises, bleeding, swelling, joint pain
- Spontaneous hemorrhage (severe cases), often in the joints but can be anywhere in the body
- Epistaxis, mucosal bleeding
- First symptoms often occur during infancy when the child becomes active, resulting in frequent bruises

Management:

- Desmopressin acetate parenterally or nasally to stimulate production of clotting factor (mild cases)
- Infusions of clotting factor from donated blood or recombinant clotting factors (genetically engineered), utilizing guidelines for dosing
- Infusions of plasma (Type C)

THALASSEMIA

Thalassemia is an inherited, autosomal recessive, thrombocytic disorder in which synthesis of one of the chains of hemoglobin (Hgb) is defective. The abnormal hemoglobin results in destruction of red blood cell membranes, aberrant RBC production, and hemolysis. The disease is classified in terms of increasing severity as thalassemia minor, intermedia, or major, with the need for chronic transfusion of RBCs increasing with severity. Thalassemia is also defined in terms of the affected hemoglobin chains and number of gene alterations. Hgb is made up of two alpha and two beta chains. If the alpha chain is defective, the person has alpha-thalassemia, which can be further differentiated as alpha trait, alpha-thalassemia minor, or Hgb H disease, depending on whether there are one, two, or three gene changes. Of these, only Hgb H disease leads to chronic hemolytic anemia. Defects in the beta chain manifest as beta-thalassemia minor (one chain, generally asymptomatic) or the much more severe, generally life-shortening beta-thalassemia major, in which beta chains are very reduced or missing and patients present with severe anemia, growth problems, jaundice, etc. Management entails transfusion, supplementation with folate and iron-chelating agents, and splenectomy.

THROMBOCYTOPENIA

Thrombocytopenia is a deficiency of circulating platelets in the blood. It can be caused by a decrease in the production of platelets from the bone marrow or an increase in destruction of platelets. Thrombocytopenia may also be caused from the use of heparin. Heparin induced thrombocytopenia can occur after heparin therapy (average 4-14 days post therapy) and is characterized by a decrease in platelet count to less than 50% of baseline or the occurrence of an unexplained thrombolytic event. A decreased production of platelets within the bone marrow can occur as a result of malignancy, bone marrow failure, infection, alcohol abuse, or a nutritional deficiency. An increase in the destruction of platelets may occur in disseminated intravascular coagulation, vasculitis, thrombotic thrombocytopenic purpura, sepsis, or idiopathic thrombocytopenic purpura.

Signs and symptoms: Signs and symptoms may include petechiae, ecchymosis, bleeding from the mouth or gums, epistaxis, pallor, weakness, fatigue, splenomegaly, blood in the urine or stool, and jaundice.

Diagnosis: Physical exam and lab studies including complete blood count, partial thromboplastin time and prothrombin time may be used to diagnosis thrombocytopenia. A bone marrow biopsy may be indicated to determine the cause of the decreased production of platelets.

Management: Treatment of thrombocytopenia involves identifying and treating the underlying cause. Medications that decrease the platelet count should be held. Platelet transfusions may be administered to patients with extremely low counts (less than 50,000) or if spontaneous bleeding occurs. Platelet transfusions are contraindicated in patients with thrombotic thrombocytopenia purpura.

HEPARIN-INDUCED THROMBOCYTOPENIA (HIT)

Heparin-induced thrombocytopenia and thrombosis syndrome (HITTS) occurs in patients receiving heparin for anticoagulation. There are two types:

- **Type I** is a transient condition occurring within a few days and causing depletion of platelets (<100,000 mm^3), but heparin may be continued as the condition usually resolves without intervention.
- **Type II** is an autoimmune reaction to heparin that occurs in 3-5% of those receiving unfractionated heparin and also occurs with low-molecular-weight heparin. It is characterized by low platelets (<50,000 mm^3) that are ≥50% below baseline. Onset is 5-14 days but can occur within hours of heparinization. Death rates are <30%. Heparin-antibody complexes form and release platelet factor 4 (PF4), which attracts heparin molecules and adheres to platelets and endothelial lining, stimulating thrombin and platelet clumping. This puts the patient at risk for thrombosis and vessel occlusion rather than hemorrhage, causing stroke, myocardial infarction, and limb ischemia with symptoms associated with the site of thrombosis. Treatment includes:
  - Discontinuation of heparin
  - Direct thrombin inhibitors (lepirudin, argatroban)
  - Monitor for signs/symptoms of thrombus/embolus

THROMBOTIC AND IDIOPATHIC THROMBOCYTOPENIC PURPURA

Thrombotic thrombocytopenic purpura (TTP) is the swift amassing of thrombi in small blood vessels subsequent to various factors such as infection, estrogen or drug use, pregnancy, or autoimmune diseases. Thrombocytopenia, low platelet counts, and hemolytic anemia are hallmark clinical and diagnostic signs. Diagnosis is also indicated by elevated lactic dehydrogenase (LDH) with normal coagulation tests. Many clinical symptoms are analogous to other conditions, for example, weakness, fever, paleness, petechiae, headache, and confusion. Other symptoms include paresis on one side, seizures, abdominal tenderness from pancreatitis, and renal failure. Management tools for TTP include antiplatelet, corticosteroid, and immunosuppressive drugs; plasmapheresis; plasma exchange; and spleen removal.

Idiopathic thrombocytopenic purpura (ITP) is an autoimmune disease in which specific IgG autoantibodies attach to platelets. The characteristic features are thrombocytopenia and bleeding or local evidence of it. ITP is typically treated with corticosteroids and, eventually, splenectomy.

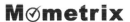

PHARMACOLOGICAL INTERVENTIONS
DRUGS FOR TREATING VASCULAR AND HEMATOLOGIC DISORDERS

The drug classifications that might be used for treatment of vascular or hematologic disorders include anticoagulants, antiplatelet agents, thrombolytic agents, and colony-stimulating factors. Anticoagulants are used for the prevention and treatment of deep vein thrombosis and pulmonary embolisms, as well as during atrial fibrillation, acute coronary syndrome, and myocardial infarction. All of these agents can cause excessive bleeding, which the physical therapist assistant should monitor. Deep tissue massage is contraindicated. Anticoagulants include coumarin derivatives, direct thrombin inhibitors, factor X_a inhibitors, and various types of heparin. Coumarin derivatives, mainly warfarin (Coumadin), impede synthesis of vitamin K-dependent clotting factors. Direct thrombin inhibitors, such as bivalirudin, directly impede thrombin. Fondaparinux (Arixtra) is a selective inhibitor of factor X_a. It can cause the adverse effect of thrombocytopenia as can heparins. Heparins extend clotting time by inhibiting the conversion of prothrombin to thrombin; they include heparin sodium and low-molecular-weight heparins (LMWHs), such as dalteparin sodium, which lessen the possibility of heparin-induced thrombocytopenia.

ANTIPLATELET AGENTS

Antiplatelet agents are indicated for the prevention of coronary heart disease, stroke, peripheral arterial disease, thrombosis associated with stent placement, and during acute coronary syndrome (with anticoagulants). These agents can increase bleeding. There are various classifications of antiplatelet agents based on their mechanism of action: glycoprotein IIb/IIIa inhibitors, cyclooxygenase inhibitors, and thienopyridines.

- **Glycoprotein IIb/IIIa inhibitors** block the receptors on platelets that bind various associated ligands, ultimately preventing platelet aggregation and thrombus formation. Examples of this class are abciximab and eptifibatide.
- **Salicylates**, delivered as **aspirin** alone or in combination with dipyridamole, act by inhibiting cyclooxygenase and prostaglandin synthetase; this impedes formation of thromboxane A_2 and platelet clumping.
- **Thienopyridines** such as **clopidogrel** (Plavix), block ADP receptors and subsequent fibrinogen binding, lessening the probability of platelet adhesion and aggregation.

THROMBOLYTICS AND COLONY-STIMULATING FACTORS

Thrombolytics (fibrinolytics) are indicated in situations where clotting is an issue, including acute coronary syndrome, ischemic stroke, critical pulmonary embolism, and catheter use. These drugs promote fibrinolysis by binding to fibrin and transforming plasminogen into plasmin. Examples of fibrinolytics are alteplase, streptokinase, and urokinase. The risk of bleeding at various sites with these agents, especially intracranially, warrants cautious use and generally abstention from physical therapy.

Colony-stimulating factors (CSF) are indicated when formation of white and red blood cells is needed. There are two classifications: those that stimulate erythropoiesis and those that stimulate granulocyte production. Erythropoiesis-stimulating factors, such as darbepoetin alpha (Aranesp) and epoetin alpha (Epogen), promote division and differentiation of erythroid progenitor cells and encourage bone marrow release of reticulocytes into the circulation where they can mature into erythrocytes. Granulocyte-stimulating factors provoke development and activation of granulocytes, either neutrophils (filgrastim) or eosinophils, monocytes, and macrophages (sargramostim). All CSFs can produce hypertension, edema, and a variety of untoward effects.

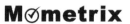

GOALS OF ANTICOAGULATION THERAPY

The goal of coagulation therapy is the achievement of a specific INR range. INR refers to the International Normalized Ratio for prothrombin time (PT). Typically, the goal range for most cardiac or vascular issues (the prevention and treatment of venous thrombosis, systemic embolisms, atrial fibrillation, etc.) is an INR between 2.0 and 3.0. For acute myocardial infarction or heart valve replacement, the goal INR range is 2.5-3.5. However, PT/INR and PTT goals should be determined by the clinician and patient-specific. Low or subtherapeutic values of PT/INR or PTT put the patient at risk for thrombus formation, while high or super-therapeutic ones can result in bleeding. The anticoagulants of choice are usually concomitant warfarin and heparin at first (or heparin alone, as it is fast-acting), followed by discontinuation of the heparin and use of warfarin alone. The physical therapist assistant should always monitor for signs of bleeding in patients on anticoagulation therapy.

BLOOD TRANSFUSIONS

Blood components that are commonly used for transfusions include:

- **Packed red blood cells**: RBCs (250-300 mL per unit) should be warmed >30 °C (optimal 37 °C) before administration to prevent hypothermia and may be reconstituted in 50-100 mL of normal saline to facilitate administration. RBCs are necessary if blood loss is about 30% (1,500-2,000 mL lost; Hgb ≤7). Above 30% blood loss, whole blood may be more effective. RBCs are most frequently used for transfusions.
- **Platelet concentrates**: Transfusions of platelets are used if the platelet count is <50,000 cells/mm^3. One unit increases the platelet count by 5,000-10,000 cells/mm^3. Platelet concentrates pose a risk for sensitization reactions and infectious diseases. Platelet concentrate is stored at a higher temperature (20-24 °C) than RBCs. This contributes to bacterial growth, so it is more prone to bacterial contamination than other blood products and may cause sepsis. Temperature increase within 6 hours should be considered an indication of possible sepsis. ABO compatibility should be observed but is not required.
- **Fresh frozen plasma** (FFP) (obtained from a unit of whole blood frozen ≤6 hours after collection) includes all clotting factors and plasma proteins, so each unit administered increases clotting factors by 2-3%. FFP may be used for deficiencies of isolated factors, excess warfarin therapy, and liver-disease-related coagulopathy. It may be used for patients who have received extensive blood transfusions but continue to hemorrhage. It is also helpful for those with antithrombin III deficiency. FFP should be warmed to 37 °C prior to administration to avoid hypothermia. ABO compatibility should be observed, if possible, but it is not required. Some patients may become sensitized to plasma proteins.
- **Cryoprecipitate** is the precipitate that forms when FFP is thawed. It contains fibrinogen, factor VIII, von Willebrand, and factor XIII. This component may be used to treat hemophilia A and hypofibrinogenemia.

ADVERSE REACTIONS

There are a number of transfusion-related complications, which is the reason that transfusions are given only when necessary. Complications include:

- **Infection**: Bacterial contamination of blood, especially platelets, can result in severe sepsis. A number of infective agents (viral, bacterial, and parasitic) can be transmitted, although increased testing of blood has decreased rates of infection markedly. Infective agents include HIV, hepatitis C and B, human T-cell lymphotropic virus, CMV, WNV, malaria, Chagas' disease, and variant Creutzfeldt-Jacob disease (from contact with mad cow disease).

- **Transfusion-related acute lung injury (TRALI)**: This respiratory distress syndrome occurs ≤6 hours after transfusion. The cause is believed to be antileukocytic or anti-HLA antibodies in the transfusion. It is characterized by non-cardiogenic pulmonary edema (high protein level) with severe dyspnea and arterial hypoxemia. Transfusion must be stopped immediately and the blood bank notified. TRALI may result in fatality but usually resolves in 12-48 hours with supportive care.
- **Graft vs. host disease**: Lymphocytes cause an immune response in immunocompromised individuals. Lymphocytes may be inactivated by irradiation, as leukocyte filters are not reliable.
- **Post-transfusion purpura**: Platelet antibodies develop and destroy the patient's platelets, so the platelet count decreases about 1 week after transfusion.
- **Transfusion-related immunosuppression**: Cell-mediated immunity is suppressed, so the patient is at increased risk of infection, and in cancer patients, transfusions may correlate with tumor recurrence. This condition relates to transfusions that include leukocytes. RBCs cause a less pronounced immunosuppression, suggesting a causative agent is in the plasma. Leukoreduction is becoming more common to reduce transmission of leukocyte-related viruses.
- **Hypothermia**: This may occur if blood products are not heated. Oxygen utilization is halved for each 10 °C decrease in normal body temperature.

VASCULAR SURGICAL PROCEDURES

Common vascular surgical procedures include embolization therapy, transcatheter thrombolysis, thrombectomy, peripheral vascular bypass grafting, and endarterectomy:

- **Embolization therapy** is the deliberate occlusion of a vessel via a catheter, usually because of improper blood flow or hemoptysis.
- **Transcatheter thrombolysis** is the direct infusion of thrombolytic agents through a catheter into a blood clot in an obstructed vessel; its best use is for acute thrombotic arterial occlusions.
- **Thrombectomy** utilizes a contact catheter placed against a vessel wall and another non-contact device that dispenses a pressurized fluid to disintegrate the clot, which is then extracted.
- In **peripheral vascular bypass grafting**, an area of vascular occlusion is bypassed using part of one of the saphenous (major leg) veins or a synthetic material, such as Gore-Tex. Patients need monitoring as they can take up to two days to become hemodynamically stable and are prone to many complications, such as site bleeding, renal failure, and thrombosis.
- In **aneurysm repair and reconstruction**, the aneurysm is clamped off on either side, excised, and interchanged with a synthetic graft.
- **Endarterectomy** is the excision of a stenotic region of an arterial wall followed by surgical reunion.

Vascular Physical Therapy Interventions

POST-VASCULAR SURGERY PHYSICAL THERAPY

Incisions made during vascular surgery should be examined before initiating physical therapy as they can drain or weep during activity, necessitating compression and/or stabilization prior to physical therapy interventions. As pulmonary infections are common in patients with abdominal and other painful incisions, the therapist should use techniques to prevent these infections, such as assisted coughing and manual procedures. Vital signs must be monitored prior to, during, and after activity as postoperative systolic blood pressures generally need to be maintained within a range that does not reduce perfusion (BP too low) or damage the graft (BP too high). Diminished distal peripheral pulses are problematic and should be reported to the nurse and physician. The physical therapist should take direction from the physician in terms of the extent of weight bearing allowed on the affected extremity, and then share this information with the physical therapist assistant. Grafting done in the hip joint area may restrict hip flexion.

PHYSICAL THERAPY FOR VASCULAR AND HEMATOLOGIC DISORDERS

The goal of physical therapy is optimization of functional mobility and activity tolerance within the context of the patient's disease-related limitations. Patients with peripheral vascular disease usually have other issues, such as coronary artery disease, diabetes, chronic obstructive lung disease, impaired sensation, renal insufficiency or failure, heart failure, venous insufficiency, liver disease, aortic dissection, and others. The therapist must be familiar with each of these conditions and how they might impact therapy. At rest and during interventions, vital signs (blood pressure, heart rate, oxygen saturation, respiratory rate) must be constantly monitored, and blood work, particularly CBCs and coagulation profiles, should be performed daily. The laboratory data should be taken into account as physical therapy may need to be deferred or modified. If values indicate risk of bleeding (low platelets, high INR) in a patient with a hematologic disorder, allowable activity levels are related to fall and hemorrhage prevention. Similarly for patients with vascular diseases, edema management (for example, through compression) and measures to deter thrombus formation are the most important considerations.

Pulmonary Physical Therapy Data Collection

ANATOMY OF THE RESPIRATORY SYSTEM

The **upper respiratory system** consists of the nose, pharynx, and larynx. The nose is comprised of two nasal cavities lined with mucous membranes and supported by bone and cartilage. It is the channel through which air enters and where that air is filtered, warmed, and humidified. At the back of the nasal cavity is the pharynx, which connects the nasal and oral cavities to the larynx and the oral cavity to the esophagus. It serves as a conduit for both air and food. At the bottom of the upper respiratory tract is the larynx, or passageway between the pharynx and trachea; it is responsible for voice production and stops food from entering the lower respiratory tract.

The **lower respiratory system** consists of the trachea and various parts of the bronchial tree. The trachea is a flexible tube made of cartilage where inspired air is cleaned, warmed, and moistened. The trachea divides into the left and right main stem bronchi of the bronchial tree within the two lungs. The bronchial tree branches into smaller secondary and tertiary bronchi and, ultimately, the bronchioles, which terminate in alveoli, tiny sacs were gas exchange occurs. Both lungs are covered with serous membranes called pleurae.

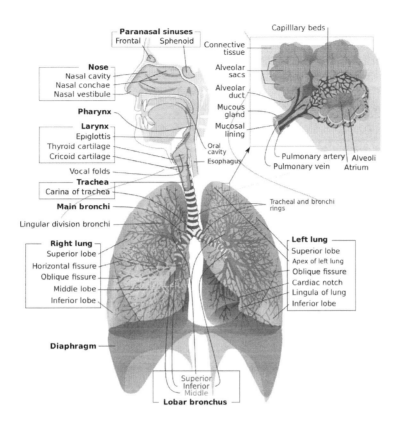

PULMONARY CIRCULATION

Pulmonary circulation is the flow of blood from the heart to the lungs. It is initiated when deoxygenated blood in the right ventricle is expelled into the pulmonary artery. The pulmonary artery divides into right and left branches, then smaller arteries, narrower arterioles, and eventually even narrower pulmonary capillaries within each lung. These pulmonary capillaries are surrounded by alveoli, which are small air sacs in the lung. The blood becomes oxygenated in the pulmonary capillaries through gas exchange, in which carbon dioxide (CO_2) is expelled and oxygen (O_2) is taken in. The oxygenated blood flows from the capillaries via the pulmonary veins into the left atrium of the heart.

MUSCLES OF INSPIRATION AND EXPIRATION

Muscles used for inspiration and expiration are separated into primary and secondary muscle groups.

- The **primary muscle groups** are those that are used in normal, quiet breathing. When patients are in respiratory distress and breathing is more difficult, secondary muscle groups become activated. The muscles considered primary for breathing are the diaphragm and the external intercostal muscles. These muscles act by changing the pressure gradient, allowing the lungs to expand and air to flow in and out.

- The **secondary muscle groups** include the sternocleidomastoid, scaleni, internal intercostals, obliques, and abdominal muscles. These secondary muscle groups work when breathing is difficult, both in inspiration and expiration, in cases such as obstructions or bronchoconstriction. Use of these secondary muscle groups can often be seen on exam and may be described as see-saw or abdominal breathing (when the abdominal muscles are being used during exhalation) or retractions as the muscles activate and can be seen between rigid structures such as bone.

ANATOMICAL LANDMARKS FOR THE LUNGS

The thorax is the upper part of the torso. It contains the lungs and heart, is divided vertically by the sternum or breastbone, and is enclosed by 12 pairs of ribs. The top seven ribs are true ribs that are connected to the sternum by costal cartilage and articulate with thoracic vertebrae. The remaining five are actually considered false ribs, as ribs 8-10 are just attached via cartilage to rib 7 and ribs 11 and 12 are merely floating. The two lungs are different in appearance from the front. The right lung has three lobes or divisions, the right upper lobe extending from the collarbone down, the right middle lobe essentially below it, and a low, outer portion called the right lower lobe. The left lung has only two lobes, the left upper lobe, approximately equivalent to the combined upper and middle portions of the right lung, and the left lower lobe. For both lungs, the posterior view only shows upper and lower lobes for each.

NEURAL CONTROL OF RESPIRATORY FUNCTIONS

Involuntary, rhythmic breathing is regulated by the medullary respiratory center in the brain stem. Respiratory rate and depth are controlled by the pneumotaxic center in the pons area of the brain. Voluntary breathing is directed by the cerebral cortex, which sends messages via motor neurons to respiratory muscles. Respiration is also under chemical control, principally the arterial levels (pressures) of oxygen (PO_2) and carbon dioxide (PCO_2) and the concentration of hydrogen ions (H^+). Respiratory rate will increase or decrease as carbon dioxide or oxygen levels respectively increase. Respiratory rate and depth can change in response to irritants or stressors.

PROCESSES INVOLVED IN PULMONARY PHYSIOLOGY

Pulmonary physiology involves ventilation, respiration, diffusion, and perfusion. Ventilation is the flow of air into and out of the lungs. Respiration is the act of breathing, which is basically related to pressure changes in the thorax and the difference between atmospheric and alveolar pressure. Inspiration occurs when the alveolar pressure is less than the atmospheric pressure, and expiration occurs when the alveolar pressure is greater than the atmospheric. The process of diffusion takes place at the alveolar-capillary membrane, where inspired oxygen (O_2) can diffuse into the bloodstream and, conversely, carbon dioxide (CO_2) can be taken in due to a concentration gradient. Perfusion is the transfer of dissolved gases between the lungs and blood cells via the cardiovascular system. Gas exchange is optimal when the ventilation/perfusion ratio (V/Q) is close to 1:1. Oxygen is ultimately transferred from the lungs to bodily tissue, about 97% through chemical combination with hemoglobin and about 3% dissolved in plasma.

PATIENT HISTORY

A respiratory evaluation should consist of patient history, physical examination, and analysis of certain specific diagnostic tests. The patient history should contain information relevant to respiratory evaluation, namely smoking history, use of oxygen therapy at rest and/or during activity, history of dyspnea (shortness of breath) at rest and/or during activity, any use-assisted or mechanical ventilation, documentation of episodes of pneumonia, and notation of thoracic procedures and other surgeries. The patient history should also document factors, such as environmental and occupational exposure to asbestos or other toxins, notation of activity level prior to admission, history of baseline sputum production, and the patient's sleeping position and number of pillows.

PULMONARY DATA COLLECTION

The data collection process for a patient undergoing evaluation for respiratory issues should include five parts: inspection, auscultation, palpation, mediate percussion, and cough examination. A meticulous inspection of the patient should examine factors, such as appearance, alertness, phonation, carriage and chest shape, skin color, notation of use of supplemental O_2 or other medical interventions, and the presence of digital clubbing or surgical incisions. In addition, a large element of the inspection should be observation of the patient's respiratory pattern for rate, depth, inspiration/expiration ratio, the succession of chest wall movements, the way different muscles appear to be used, and the general ease of breathing. A normal respiratory rate is 12-20 breaths per minute, and the customary inspiration/expiration ratio is one or two.

AUSCULTATION FOR BREATH SOUNDS

For respiratory evaluation, the clinician uses auscultation (the use of a stethoscope) to listen for normal, abnormal, and adventitious breath sounds, as well as extrapulmonary sounds and voice sounds. The clinician uses the flat diaphragm of the stethoscope to hear sounds on the anterior, lateral, and posterior portions of both lungs. The patient, who is seated or prone, breathes through the mouth.

Normal breath sounds can be divided into three types.

- **Vesicular breath sounds** are low, soft sounds that can normally be heard over the peripheral lung space.
- **Bronchovesicular breath sounds** are moderate pitch breath sounds that are normally heard in the upper lung fields.
- **Tracheal breath sounds** are higher in pitch and heard over the trachea.

Abnormal breath sounds are also known as adventitious lung sounds.

- **Wheezes** are high-pitched, expiratory sounds caused by air flowing through an obstructed airway.
- **Stridor** is also high-pitched, but is usually heard on inspiration in the upper airways.
- **Coarse crackles** are caused by an excessive amount of secretions in the airway and can be heard on inspiration and expiration.
- **Fine crackles** occur late in the expiratory phase and usually occur when the peripheral airways are being "popped" back open.

> **Review Video: Lung Sounds**
> Visit mometrix.com/academy and enter code: 765616

AUSCULTATION FOR VOICE SOUNDS

Voice sounds, or phonation, can be heard with an intensity related to the area of the bronchial tree, just as with breath sounds. Voice sound tests with auscultation corroborate breath sound findings. Three kinds of voice sound tests are suggested. The first is whispered pectoriloquy, in which the individual whispers "one, two, three." If these sounds can be heard in distal lung areas, there is consolidation present, and if they are barely audible in distal portions, then hyperinflation is indicated. A similar test is bronchophony, in which the patient repeatedly says the phrase "ninety-nine"; indications are the same as for pectoriloquy. The third suggested voice sound test is

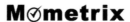

egophony, in which the person repeats the letter "e" during auscultation; if it sounds like "a" in the distal areas, then the presence of fluid in the lung parenchyma or air spaces is implied.

PALPATION

During respiratory evaluation, palpation, or medical examination using finger pressure, should be performed on the upper, middle, and lower lung fields. The clinician faces the patient and uses the thumb and fingers on both hands to palpate near the collarbone, in the middle of the chest, and slightly lower, respectively. They should note whether there is fremitus or vibrations during respiration; these occur during voice production but also indicate the presence of secretions. Palpation should also be used to elucidate areas and reproducibility of pain or tenderness, skin temperature, pattern of chest expansion, existence of rib fractures and/or bony anomalies, and the presence of subcutaneous emphysema. The latter results from air in subcutaneous tissues due to pneumothorax, poor central line placement, or thoracic surgery, and manifests during palpation as bubbles that pop.

MEDIATE PERCUSSION

Mediate percussion is a technique in which a clinician places the palm side of the index and/or middle finger along an intercostal space in the chest wall and then uses the tips of the index and/or middle finger of the other hand to thump against the tip of the finger resting on the chest wall. The front and back areas of the chest are thus evaluated. The sounds heard during mediate percussion are characteristic; normal lung tissue should sound resonant. Possible abnormalities include sounds that are hyper resonant, indicating emphysema or pneumothorax; tympanic or vibrating, if there is abdominal gas; dull when there is decreased air in the lungs or dense tissues; and flat or very dull in areas of extremely dense tissue. Mediate percussion is also used to determine the position of the diaphragm during regular and deep breathing and the relative shift, or diaphragmatic excursion, on each side of the posterior chest wall.

COUGH EXAMINATION

Cough examination involves either instructing the patient to cough or observing as they naturally cough. Coughing should consist of four stages, each of which must be seen. Normally, the first phase is full inspiration, followed by the second, closure of the glottis accompanied by augmented intrathoracic pressure. The third phase is the abdominal contraction, and the final is the quick expulsion of air. If any step is not done properly, pulmonary secretion clearance is impacted. During cough examination, the clinician should observe the patient for the effectiveness of secretion clearance, capacity to control coughing, the quality of clearance (wet, dry, or spastic), the rate of occurrence, and characteristics of the sputum, including presence of hemoptysis (the expectoration of blood).

PULSE OXIMETRY

Pulse oximetry is a technique in which finger or ear sensors detect arterial oxyhemoglobin saturation (SaO_2). The oxyhemoglobin saturation is related to the partial pressure of oxygen (PaO_2) fairly linearly until high saturation is achieved. Thus, pulmonary reserve and the possibility of hypoxia, or oxygen deprivation, can be indirectly determined using pulse oximetry. Normal oxyhemoglobin saturation is usually of 95-100% and corresponds to 90-100 mmHg oxygen partial pressure. Some patients, such as those with COPD, may have a normal oxygen saturation of 88-92%. Otherwise, an SaO_2 of less 90% or PaO_2 of less than 60 mmHg require supplemental oxygen and present symptomatically as tachypnea and/or tachycardia.

PULMONARY LABORATORY TESTS
ARTERIAL BLOOD GAS ANALYSIS

Arterial blood gases (ABGs) are monitored to assess effectiveness of oxygenation, ventilation, and acid-base status and to determine oxygen flow rates. Partial pressure of a gas is that exerted by each gas in a mixture of gases, proportional to its concentration, based on total atmospheric pressure of 760 mmHg at sea level. Normal values include:

- Acidity/alkalinity (pH): 7.35-7.45
- Partial pressure of carbon dioxide ($PaCO_2$): 35-45 mmHg
- Partial pressure of oxygen (PaO_2): ≥80 mmHg
- Bicarbonate concentration (HCO_3^-): 22-26 mEq/L
- Oxygen saturation (SaO_2): ≥95%

The relationship between these elements, particularly the $PaCO_2$ and the PaO_2 indicates respiratory status. For example, $PaCO_2$ >55 and the PaO_2 <60 in a patient previously in good health indicates respiratory failure. There are many issues to consider. Ventilator management may require a higher $PaCO_2$ to prevent barotrauma and a lower PaO_2 to reduce oxygen toxicity.

INTERPRETATION OF ARTERIAL BLOOD GAS ANALYSIS

A patient is considered acidotic when their arterial blood gas pH is less than 7.35. Conversely, the patient is considered alkalotic when their arterial blood gas pH is higher than 7.45. Both conditions indicate an acid-base imbalance and potential an underlying respiratory or metabolic disorder that must be addressed to normalize the pH. The PCO_2 levels will be outside of normal range if the primary problem is respiratory in origin:

- A low pH in combination with a high PCO_2 suggests uncompensated **respiratory acidosis**
- A high pH along with a low PCO_2 indicates uncompensated **respiratory alkalosis**

The HCO_3 levels will be outside the normal range if the primary disorder is metabolic in origin.

- Both pH and HCO_3 are low in uncompensated **metabolic acidosis**
- Both pH and HCO_3 are high for an uncompensated **metabolic alkalosis**.

Metabolic and respiratory processes sometimes compensate for one another, in which case the HCO_3 or PCO_2 may shift toward correcting the other. The oxygen pressure or levels measured by the PO_2 are used to determine hypoxia, referring to inadequate oxygen levels of less than 80 mmHg.

PULMONARY DIAGNOSTIC TESTS
CHEST X-RAYS

Chest x-rays or radiographs are used for differential diagnosis of pulmonary states. They are useful for diagnosing and monitoring conditions such as airspace consolidation (present in a number of cardiopulmonary diseases), identifying airspaces, diagnosing lobar atelectasis or collapse, pinpointing nodules or abscesses, evaluating certain structural features, or identifying where to place tubes or lines. CXRs are generally described in terms of where the x-ray beam enters and exits, with the three most prevalent types being posterior-anterior (P-A), anterior-posterior (A-P), and lateral. The preferred position for all types is upright sitting or standing. The A-P type may be taken semi-reclined or lying down, while the lateral type might be shot as the patient lies on their side. Denser structures, such as bone, appear whiter or radiopaque on a chest x-ray; intermediate ones, like the heart and pulmonary vessels, are shades of gray; and airspaces should be relatively dark or radiolucent.

BRONCHOSCOPY

Bronchoscopy utilizes a thin, flexible fiberoptic bronchoscope to inspect the larynx, trachea, and bronchi for diagnostic purposes. It is also used to collect specimens, obtain biopsies, remove foreign bodies or secretions, treat atelectasis, and to excise lesions. The patient is in supine position during the procedure. The Mallampati classification may be used to determine difficulty of airway. The patient receives local anesthesia to the nares (lidocaine gel) and oropharynx (lidocaine gel, spray, or nebulizer), and usually receives a benzodiazepine (commonly midazolam or lorazepam), an opioid (fentanyl or meperidine), or propofol. Medications are usually given in small incremental doses throughout the procedure and may be combined. Over-sedation may cause physiologic depression, but undersedation may result in recall and agitation with sympathetic activation. The tube is advanced through the nares and down the trachea to the bronchi. Airway patency, respiratory rate, and oxygen saturation must be constantly monitored. Complications can include bleeding, arrhythmias, obstruction, laryngospasm, and respiratory failure.

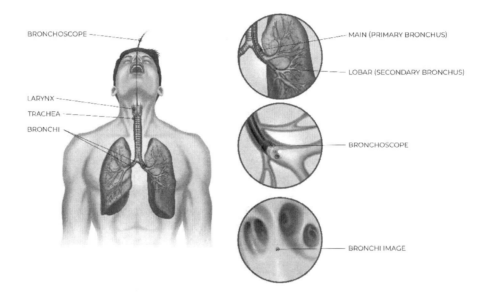

VENTILATION/PERFUSION SCANS AND CT PULMONARY ANGIOGRAPHY

Ventilation/perfusion or V/Q lung scans are done in tandem. The ventilation portion involves the inhalation of inert radioactive gases by the patient, projections are then taken after the first breath, at equilibrium, and during washout. The perfusion scan involves intravenous injection of a radioisotope, after which six projections are obtained. The perfusion portion, which distinguishes deficient blood flow, is useful for detecting a variety of pulmonary diseases or lesions, as well as hypoventilation. Comparison between ventilation and perfusion scans is done to evaluate the V/Q matching, which should be about 0.8.

Computerized tomographic pulmonary angiography (CT-PA) is a technique primarily used to visualize the pulmonary artery and find pulmonary embolisms or thrombi.

PULMONARY FUNCTION TESTS

Pulmonary function tests (PFTs) are a series of measurements of an individual's lung volumes during various phases of breathing, a number of associated capacities, and inspiratory and expiratory flow rates. PFTs are performed for reasons such as the detection and quantification of pulmonary diseases, differentiation between obstructive and restrictive lung diseases, determination of the extent of pulmonary contribution to systemic diseases, appraisal of disease progression, measurement of the response to certain respiratory therapies, and determination of the extent of impairment. Pulmonary function tests are performed using instruments that the patient breathes into, called spirometers (volume, flow, or gas dilution), or utilizing enclosed body plethysmography. Normal values are dependent on a number of factors, such as age and height, and are predicted from available nomograms (scaled graphs), or regression equations. There are quite a few types of PFTs, but the most important ones are those that indicate airway patency during expiration. These are forced expiratory volume in 1 second (FEV_1), forced vital capacity (FVC), and their ratio (FEV_1/FVC).

Pulmonary function tests measuring lung volume include:

- **Inspiratory reserve volume** (IRV): The maximum volume of air inspired with a full and forceful inspiration; a decreased value suggests obstructive pulmonary disease.
- **Expiratory reserve volume** (ERV): The maximum volume of air expired in a forceful expiration; a decreased value suggests ascites, pleural effusions, or pneumothorax.
- **Tidal volume** (TV): The volume of air taken in or breathed out during one breath while resting; a decreased value suggests restrictive lung diseases, malignancy.
- **Residual volume** (RV): The volume of air still present in lungs at the end of expiration; distinguishes between obstructive (increased RV) and restrictive (decreased RV) lung disease.
- **Total lung capacity** (TLC): The total lung volume at the conclusion of maximal inspiration; calculated as the sum of all above volumes (IRV+ ERV + TV + RV); also distinguishes between obstructive (increased) and restrictive (decreased) lung diseases.
- **Vital capacity** (VC): The maximum air volume that can be expired slowly; expressed as the sum of TV + IRV + ERV.
- **Functional residual capacity** (FRC): The air volume still in the lungs at the conclusion of normal expiration; equal to the sum of ERV + RV; indicative of obstructive (increased) versus restrictive (decreased) disease.
- **Inspiratory capacity** (IC): The largest possible inspiratory volume after resting expiration; the sum of TV + IRV; a decreased value suggests restriction.
- **RV:TLC × 100**: the relative percentage of unexpired residual volume to total lung capacity; obstructive disorders are suggested if this is greater than 35%.

PULMONARY SPIROMETRY TESTS

Pulmonary spirometry tests performed include:

- **Forced vital capacity** (FVC): Air volume is forcefully and quickly expired subsequent to maximum inspiration; usually equal to vital capacity (VC), except in obstructive diseases (decreased).
- **Forced expiratory volume timed** (FEV_t): The air volume forcefully expired during a specific time interval, generally 1 second (FEV_1), which is decreased in both obstructive and restrictive lung disorders.
- **FEV%**: The percentage of FVC expired during a specific time interval, generally 1 second, thus calculated usually as $FEV_1/FVC \times 100$; used to distinguish between obstructive (decreased) and restrictive (increased) disorders.
- **Forced expiratory flow 25-75%** ($FEF_{25-75\%}$): The average airflow in the middle of measuring FEV; indicative of peripheral airway resistance; if decreased, medium-sized airways are obstructed.
- **Peak expiratory flow rate** (PEFR): Maximal achievable airflow rate during FEV testing.

- **Maximum voluntary ventilation** (MVV): The maximal achievable air volume breathed in 1 minute voluntarily; generally calculated by measuring for 10-15 seconds and multiplying accordingly; indicative of the status of respiratory muscles, airway and tissue resistance, and lung and thorax compliance.
- **Flow-volume loop** (F-V) loop: A graphic representation of maximal FEV and maximum inspiratory flow volume.

VENTILATION TESTS AND GAS EXCHANGE TESTS

There are three types of ventilation tests:

- **Minute volume** (VE), or minute ventilation, is the entire volume of air inspired or expired in one minute. It is calculated as: VE = VT (tidal volume) × respiratory rate. VE is often measured during exercise or stress testing as it increases when the patient is hypoxic, has too much carbon dioxide in the blood, or has acidosis.
- The **respiratory dead space** (VD) is the air volume ventilated but not perfused. VD is important because it is indicative of the surface area accessible for gas exchange. More dead space means decreased gas exchange.
- **Alveolar ventilation** (VA) indicates the air volume participating in gas exchange, estimable as (VT - VD). VA estimations of oxygen availability are generally backed up with arterial blood gas measurements.

The gas exchange test performed is the diffusing capacity of carbon monoxide (DLCO), in which the patient inhales a mixture of carbon monoxide and helium. After exhaling for 10 seconds, the gases are quantified. DLCO is indicative of the gas exchange area, the extent of contact between a functioning pulmonary capillary bed and functioning alveoli.

Pulmonary Diseases/Conditions that Impact Effective Treatment

OBSTRUCTIVE VS. RESTRICTIVE LUNG DISEASE

Obstructive lung diseases or conditions are states where there is diminished airflow out of the lungs due to narrowing of the airway lumen. The general result is more dead space and decreased surface area available for gas exchange. Obstructive pulmonary conditions include asthma, chronic bronchitis, emphysema, cystic fibrosis, and bronchiectasis. Obstructive situations in which there are airflow limitations that cannot be completely reversed are collectively referred to as COPD, chronic obstructive pulmonary disease.

With **restrictive lung disease**, there is decreased lung compliance, making expansion and breathing difficult. Often the underlying issue is tissue scarring. Restrictive lung disorders include atelectasis, pneumonia, pulmonary edema, adult respiratory distress syndrome (ARDS), pulmonary embolisms (PE), and lung contusions.

CHRONIC ASTHMA

The three primary symptoms of chronic asthma are cough, wheezing, and dyspnea. In cough-variant asthma, a severe cough may be the only symptom, at least initially. Chronic asthma is characterized by recurring bronchospasm and inflammation of the airways resulting in airway obstruction. Asthma affects the bronchi and not the alveoli. While no longer considered part of COPD because airway obstruction is not constant and is responsive to treatment, over time fibrotic changes in the airways can result in permanent obstruction, especially if asthma is not treated adequately. **Symptoms** of chronic asthma include nighttime coughing, exertional dyspnea, tightness in the chest, and cough. Acute exacerbations may occur, sometimes related to triggers, such as allergies, resulting in increased dyspnea, wheezing, cough, tachycardia, bronchospasm, and rhonchi. **Management** of chronic asthma includes chest hygiene, identification and avoidance of triggers, prompt treatment of infections, bronchodilators, long-acting β-2 agonists, and inhaled glucocorticoids.

CHRONIC BRONCHITIS

Chronic bronchitis is a pulmonary airway disease characterized by severe cough with sputum production for at least 3 months a year for at least 2 consecutive years. Irritation of the airways (often from smoke or pollutants) causes an inflammatory response, increasing the number of mucus-secreting glands and goblet cells while ciliary function decreases so that the extra mucus plugs the airways. Additionally, the bronchial walls thicken, alveoli near the inflamed bronchioles become fibrotic, and alveolar macrophages cannot function properly, increasing susceptibility to infections. Chronic bronchitis is most common in those >45 years old and occurs twice as frequently in females as males.

Symptoms include:

- Persistent cough with increasing sputum
- Dyspnea
- Frequent respiratory infections

Management includes:

- Bronchodilators
- Long term continuous oxygen therapy or supplemental oxygen during exercise
- Pulmonary rehabilitation to improve exercise and breathing
- Antibiotics during infections
- Corticosteroids for acute episodes

EMPHYSEMA

Emphysema, the primary component of COPD, is characterized by abnormal distention of air spaces at the ends of the terminal bronchioles, with destruction of alveolar walls so that there is less and less gaseous exchange and increasing dead space with resultant hypoxemia, hypercapnia, and respiratory acidosis. The capillary bed is damaged as well, altering pulmonary blood flow and raising pressure in the right atrium (cor pulmonale) and pulmonary artery, leading to cardiac failure. Complications include respiratory insufficiency and failure. There are two primary types of emphysema (and both forms may be present):

- **Centrilobular** (the most common form) involves the central portion of the respiratory lobule, sparing distal alveoli, and usually affects the upper lobes. Typical symptoms include abnormal ventilation-perfusion ratios, hypoxemia, hypercapnia, and polycythemia with right-sided heart failure.
- **Panlobular** involves enlargement of all air spaces, including the bronchiole, alveolar duct, and alveoli, but there is minimal inflammatory disease. Typical symptoms include hyperextended rigid barrel chest, marked dyspnea, weight loss, and active expiration.

CYSTIC FIBROSIS

Cystic fibrosis (CF) is a hereditary disorder affecting the exocrine glands. The result is fibrosis of the pancreas and buildup of secretions in many bodily systems, including the lungs, where it is a relatively fatal obstructive lung disease. After babies with CF experience an infection, their bronchial and bronchiolar walls get inflamed; the bronchial glands and goblet cells enlarge, producing persistent secretions; and clearance of the secretions is diminished. Pulmonary abnormalities associated with CF include bronchospasm, augmented airway resistance, V/Q mismatch, and increased susceptibility to respiratory infections. CF patients display tachypnea, accessory muscle use, generalized weakness, and a barrel chest. Palpation reveals tachycardia, hypertension, and increased chest diameter, and auscultation should show diminished breath sounds, rhonchi, and crackles. Patients have a controlled or intermittent cough with very thick, greenish, possibly bloody sputum. Their chest x-rays show fibrosis, atelectasis, an enlarged right ventricle, streaks, translucent lung fields, and flattened diaphragms. They also have a dysfunctional pancreas that secretes thick mucus rather than the enzymes needed to digest food. For this reason, patients with CF require supplemental pancreatic enzymes to assist in the digestion of food. Additional management includes antibiotics, bronchodilators, mucolytics, supplemental oxygen, often lung transplantation, and other support.

BRONCHIECTASIS

Bronchiectasis is a lung disorder in which there is both obstruction and restriction. It is technically defined as the permanent expansion of larger airways (typically, those with a diameter >2 mm). The causative agents include bacterial respiratory infections, cystic fibrosis, tuberculosis, and ciliary defects. Bronchiectasis is characterized by the destruction of bronchiole walls and the mucociliary escalator; dilation, fibrosis, and ulceration of the bronchioles; and enlargement of the bronchial artery. Signs are similar to cystic fibrosis, namely tachypnea, accessory muscle use, generalized weakness, and a barrel chest. Physical examination findings are comparable to CF as well, including a rapid heart rate, hypertension, expanded chest diameter, diminished breath sounds, crackles, and rhonchi. The sputum from a bronchiectasis patient's cough is purulent, smells foul, and may contain blood. Chest x-rays reveal patchy infiltrates, often atelectasis, increased markings on blood vessels and bronchi, and, if severe, a honeycombing appearance. Treatments include antibiotics, bronchodilators, corticosteroids, supplemental oxygen, dispensation of IV fluids, bronchopulmonary hygiene, nutritional sustenance, lung transplantation, and sometimes pain medication.

ATELECTASIS

Atelectasis is a restrictive lung condition in which alveoli, one or more lung segments, or one or more lobes have collapsed partially or totally. It is usually a result of hypoventilation or unsuccessful pulmonary secretion clearance, but it can also occur for other reasons, such as after a bout of pneumonia, situations that restrict the diaphragm (e.g., paralysis), and/or the compression of lung tissue. A ventilation/perfusion mismatch, shunting, and vasoconstriction result ultimately in hypoxemia. The patient may or may not present with rapid breathing, shallow respirations, and/or fever. The main observations on palpation are a decreased tactile fremitus, vocal resonance, and sometimes a rapid heartbeat. Auscultation reveals crackles, where the atelectasis has occurred, and reduced breath sounds. If a lobe has collapsed, breath sounds are missing or bronchial. The sputum characteristics depend on the underlying cause; characteristic chest x-ray findings feature linear opaque areas at the site, fissures, displacement of the diaphragm, and, in cases of lobar collapse, a dense, white triangular area. Atelectasis is managed by using incentive spirometry, supplemental oxygen, bronchopulmonary hygiene, and mobilization.

PNEUMONIA

Pneumonia is inflammation of the lung parenchyma, filling the alveoli with exudate. It is common throughout childhood and adulthood. Pneumonia may be a primary disease or may occur secondary to another infection or disease, such as lung cancer. Pneumonia may be caused by bacteria, viruses, parasites, or fungi. Common causes for community-acquired pneumonia (CAP) include:

- Streptococcus pneumoniae
- Legionella species
- Haemophilus influenzae
- Staphylococcus aureus
- Mycoplasma pneumoniae
- Viruses

Pneumonia may also be caused by chemical damage. Pneumonia is characterized by **location**:

- **Lobar** involves one or more lobes of the lungs. If lobes in both lungs are affected, it is referred to as bilateral or double pneumonia.
- **Bronchial/lobular** involves the terminal bronchioles, and exudate can involve the adjacent lobules. Usually, the pneumonia occurs in scattered patches throughout the lungs.
- **Interstitial** involves primarily the interstitium and alveoli where white blood cells and plasma fill the alveoli, generating inflammation and creating fibrotic tissue as the alveoli are destroyed.

> **Review Video: Pneumonia**
> Visit mometrix.com/academy and enter code: 628264

PULMONARY EDEMA

Pulmonary edema, the buildup of excess fluid, is a restrictive pulmonary condition divided into two categories depending on origin: cardiogenic pulmonary edema and noncardiogenic pulmonary edema. Cardiogenic pulmonary edema is characterized by the backflow of blood from the heart (due to left ventricular hypertrophy, etc.), which encourages fluid movement from the pulmonary capillaries into the alveolar spaces. This ultimately results in fluid buildup in many areas of the bronchial tree. Capillary permeability changes can also occur subtly subsequent to other conditions, such as pneumonia or adult respiratory distress syndrome, resulting in noncardiogenic pulmonary edema. In either case, patients develop atelectasis, V/Q mismatch, and hypoxemia. Signs present as rapid breathing, anxiety, accessory muscle use, and orthopnea, which is significant because the physical therapist assistant should avoid treating these patients while supine. Physical findings include increased tactile and vocal fremitus on palpation, symmetric wet crackles, possible wheezing on auscultation, and relatively clear sputum. Chest radiographs show increased hilar vascular markings, short horizontal lines, left ventricular hypertrophy, fluffy opaque heart areas, and sometimes pleural effusion. Treatment includes diuretics, oxygen, hemodynamic monitoring, and possibly other drugs.

ACUTE RESPIRATORY DISTRESS SYNDROME

Acute lung injury (ALI) comprises a syndrome of respiratory distress culminating in acute respiratory distress syndrome (ARDS). ARDS is a dangerous, potentially fatal respiratory condition, always caused by an illness or injury to the lungs. Lung injury causes fluid to leak into the spaces between the alveoli and capillaries, increasing pressure on the alveoli, causing them to collapse. With increased fluid accumulation in the lungs, the ability of the lungs to move oxygen into the blood is decreased, resulting in hypoxemia. Lung injury also causes a release of cytokines, a type of inflammatory protein, which then brings neutrophils to the lung. These proteins and cells leak into nearby blood vessels and cause inflammation throughout the body. This immune response, in combination with low levels of blood oxygen, can lead to organ failure. Symptoms are characterized by respiratory distress within 72 hours of surgery or a serious injury to a person with otherwise normal lungs and no cardiac disorder. Untreated, the condition results in respiratory failure, MODS, and a mortality rate of 5-30%.

Symptoms include:

- Refractory hypoxemia (hypoxemia not responding to increasing levels of oxygen)
- Crackling rales/wheezing in lungs
- Decrease in pulmonary compliance which results in increased tachypnea with expiratory grunting
- Cyanosis/skin mottling
- Hypotension and tachycardia
- Symptoms associated with volume overload are missing (3rd heart sound or JVD)
- Respiratory alkalosis initially but, as the disease progresses, replaced with hypercarbia and respiratory acidosis
- Normal x-ray initially but then diffuse infiltrates in both lungs, while the heart and vessels appear normal

Management strategies include mechanical ventilation, IV fluids, homodynamic monitoring, and nitrous oxide therapy. Prone positioning can be used by experienced professionals as it allows greater aeration to dorsal segments, better V/Q matching, and improved drainage of secretions.

PULMONARY EMBOLISM

Acute pulmonary embolism occurs when a pulmonary artery or arteriole is blocked, cutting off blood supply to the pulmonary vessels and subsequent oxygenation of the blood. While most pulmonary emboli are from thrombus formation, they can also be caused by air, fat, or septic embolus (from bacterial invasion of a thrombus). Common originating sites for thrombus formation are the deep veins in the legs, the pelvic veins, and the right atrium. Causes include stasis related to damage to endothelial wall and changes in blood coagulation factors. Atrial fibrillation poses a serious risk because blood pools in the right atrium, forming clots that travel directly through the right ventricle to the lungs. The obstruction of the artery/arteriole causes an increase in alveolar dead space in which there is ventilation but impairment of gas exchange because of the ventilation/perfusion mismatching or intrapulmonary shunting. This results in hypoxia, hypercapnia, and the release of mediators that cause bronchoconstriction. If more than 50% of the vascular bed becomes excluded, pulmonary hypertension occurs.

Physical examination shows hypotension, rapid heart rate, locally decreased chest wall expansion, wheezing, crackles, and diminished or missing breath sounds distal to the embolism. A chest radiograph should display decreased lung volume, a dilated pulmonary artery with markings, and possibly atelectasis and/or density at the infarct location with distal radiolucency. Therapies include anticoagulation measures, hemodynamic stabilization, oxygen, mechanical ventilation, thrombolysis, embolectomy, and filters inserted into the inferior vena cava. Physical therapy should not be performed during a confirmed or suspected PE.

INTERSTITIAL LUNG DISEASE AND LUNG CONTUSIONS

These are two types of restrictive lung disease: interstitial lung disease and lung contusion. Interstitial lung disease (ILD) is the universal name for any condition in which respiratory membranes in many areas of the lung are destroyed through inflammation and fibrosis. There are many potential causes of ILD, and the main observed symptom is dyspnea upon exertion.

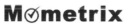

Lung contusion is a situation in which some type of trauma initially causes lung tissue to compress against the chest wall producing a rupture at the alveolar-capillary membrane with subsequent hemorrhaging. Decompression then follows, stretching the tissues. Blood and fluid buildup in the alveoli and interstitial areas, causing shunting and other problems, with an end result of hypoxemia. Patients present with tachypnea, bleeding along the chest wall, and cyanosis, if advanced. Physical examination reveals hypotension, tachycardia, crackling noises due to broken ribs, diminished or missing breath sounds at the site, wet crackles, and sometimes a weak cough with relatively clear sputum. CXR shows patchy but localized opacities and consolidation, if present. Lung contusions are treated with pain management, oxygen, mechanical ventilation, and IV fluids.

PLEURAL EFFUSION

Pleural effusion is the accumulation of fluid in the pleural space, usually secondary to other disease processes, such as heart failure, TB, neoplasms, nephrotic syndrome, and viral respiratory infections. The fluid may be serous, bloody, or purulent (empyema) and transudative or exudative. Signs and symptoms depend on underlying condition but includes dyspnea, from mild to severe. Tracheal deviation away from affected side may be evident. Diagnosis includes chest x-ray, lateral decubitus x-ray, CT, thoracentesis, and pleural biopsy. Treatment includes treating underlying cause, thoracentesis to remove fluid, insertion of chest tube, pleurodesis, or pleurectomy or pleuroperitoneal shunt (primarily with malignancy).

> **Review Video: Pleural Effusions**
> Visit mometrix.com/academy and enter code: 145719

PNEUMOTHORAX

Pneumothorax occurs when there is a leak of air into the pleural space, resulting in complete or partial collapse of a lung.

Symptoms: Vary widely depending on the cause and degree of the pneumothorax and whether or not there is an underlying disease. Symptoms include acute pleuritic pain (95%), usually on the affected side, and decreased breath sounds. In a *tension pneumothorax,* symptoms include tracheal deviation and hemodynamic compromise.

Diagnosis: Clinical findings; radiograph: 6-foot upright posterior-anterior; ultrasound may detect traumatic pneumothorax.

Management: Chest-tube thoracostomy with underwater seal drainage is the most common treatment for all types of pneumothorax.

- Tension pneumothorax: Immediate needle decompression and chest tube thoracostomy
- Small pneumothorax, patient stable: Oxygen administration and observation for 3-6 hours. If no increase is shown on repeat x-ray, patient may be discharged with another x-ray in 24 hours.
- Primary spontaneous pneumothorax: Catheter aspiration or chest tube thoracostomy

PNEUMOTHORAX

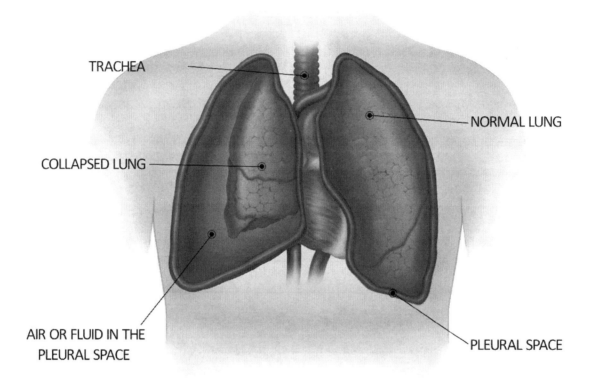

TRACHEA

NORMAL LUNG

COLLAPSED LUNG

AIR OR FLUID IN THE PLEURAL SPACE

PLEURAL SPACE

HEMOTHORAX, EMPYEMA, AND FLAIL CHEST

Hemothorax is the existence of blood in the pleural space due to some type of injury to the pleura. It presents symptomatically, through physical findings, and on chest radiographs very similarly to pneumothorax, air in the pleural space. If there is associated lung contusion, hemoptysis (the coughing up of blood) can distinguish it from pneumothorax. Management strategies include supplemental oxygen, chest tube placement, pain control if needed, and blood transfusions. Patients with hemothorax should be monitored for shock and treated, if necessary. Hemopneumothorax means there is both blood and air in the pleural space.

Empyema is a pleural effusion in which the collection of pleural fluid is thick and purulent, usually as a result of bacterial pneumonia or penetrating chest trauma. Empyema may also occur as a complication of thoracentesis or thoracic surgery. Signs and symptoms include acute illness with fever, chills, pain, cough, and dyspnea. Diagnosis is per chest CT and thoracentesis with culture and

72

sensitivity. Treatment includes antibiotics and drainage of pleural space per needle aspiration, tube thoracostomy, or open chest drainage with thoracotomy.

A **flail chest** is a situation in which three or more contiguous ribs are broken due to some type of chest injury or forceful cardiopulmonary resuscitation. Changes in pressure gradients cause paradoxical breathing where the ribs move in opposition to normal patterns, there is contused lung tissue underneath, and mediastinal shifting may occur.

BREATHING ABNORMALITIES AND DEFECTS

Specific breathing abnormalities and the associated defects include:

- **Apnea**: No airflow to the lungs for longer than 15 seconds due to airway obstruction, cardiopulmonary arrest, or narcotic overdose.
- **Bradypnea**: Less than 12 breaths per minute due to sedative or alcohol use, fatigue, or certain neurologic or metabolic disorders.
- **Tachypnea**: More than 20 breaths per minute, usually resulting from acute respiratory distress, anemia, etc.

Respiratory depth abnormalities include:

- **Hyperpnea**: Increased depth of breathing associated with congestive heart failure (CHF), pulmonary infections, or activity.
- **Cheyne-Stokes respirations**: Increasing depth of breathing followed by a phase of apnea due to CHF, narcotic overdose, or elevated intracranial pressure.

Combined or paradoxical abnormalities include:

- **Hyperventilation**: Rate and depth increased with depressed PCO_2 due to anxiety or metabolic acidosis.
- **Hypoventilation**: Rate and depth decreased with increased PCO_2 due to metabolic alkalosis or anything that depresses respiration, such as sedation or overmedication.
- **Biot's respirations**: Depth of breath increased followed by a phase of apnea; due to high intracranial pressure or meningitis.
- **Kussmaul's respirations**: Higher but regular rate and depth; due to diabetic ketoacidosis or renal failure.
- **Orthopnea**: Dyspnea while lying down, generally due to chronic lung disease or CHF.
- **Paradoxical respirations**: Abdominal or chest wall moves in upon inspiration and out upon expiration; due to paralysis or trauma.
- **Sighing respirations**: Sighing more than two to three times a minute; associated with dyspnea, angina, or fear.

TYPES OF RESPIRATORY DYSFUNCTION

Types of respiratory dysfunction include:

- **Hypoxemia and hypoxia**: Low levels of oxygen in the blood and tissues, respectively.
- **Air trapping**: Retention of gas in the lung due to airway obstruction.
- **Bronchospasm**: The contraction of smooth muscle in the walls of bronchi and bronchioles, causing constriction.
- **Consolidation**: Replacement of alveolar air with transudate, exudate, or tissue fragments.
- **Hyperinflation**: Overexpansion of the lungs at rest due to air trapping.

73

- **Respiratory distress**: A condition in which inadequate gas exchange causes a combination of shortness of breath, respiratory muscle fatigue, aberrant respiratory pattern and rate, nervousness, and cyanosis; usually leads to respiratory failure if untreated.
- **Respiratory failure**: Incapacity of respiratory system to maintain adequate oxygen-carbon dioxide gas exchange

ACID-BASE IMBALANCES

Acid-base imbalances, as measured by arterial blood gas analysis, are a result of an underlying respiratory or metabolic dysfunction. Patients with acidosis have a pH of less than 7.35, while those with alkalosis have a pH higher than approximately 7.45.

- **Respiratory acidosis** can be caused by chronic obstructive pulmonary disease (COPD), pneumothorax (air in the pleural cavity), pulmonary edema, or trauma to the chest wall. It can also result from less obvious sources, such as sedation, drug overdose, head trauma, sleep apnea, or central nervous system disorders in which ventilation of CO_2 is insufficient, and a buildup occurs.
- **Metabolic acidosis** often results from lactic acidosis or ketoacidosis. The latter may be attributed to diabetes, diarrhea, starvation, alcohol abuse, or use of parenteral nutrition. It can also result from the retention of toxins resulting from renal failure.
- **Respiratory alkalosis** results from hyperventilation due to a pulmonary embolism, hypoxia, pulmonary edema, asthma, or acute respiratory distress syndrome, as well as less obvious issues like anxiety, pregnancy, sepsis, and fever. The condition is also indicative of congestive heart failure (CHF).
- **Metabolic alkalosis** results from the excessive loss of acid, often due to vomiting, the use of diuretics or steroids, or nasogastric suction. It can also result from low blood potassium, ingestion of excessive amounts of antacids, excessive administration of bicarbonate, Cushing's syndrome, or blood transfusions.

PULMONARY PHARMACOLOGICAL INTERVENTIONS
PHARMACOLOGIC INTERVENTIONS FOR ASTHMA

Numerous pharmacological agents are used for control of asthma, some that are long-acting to prevent attacks and others that are short-acting to provide relief for acute episodes. Listed with each are the standard medications and dosage used for urgent care:

- **β-Adrenergic agonists** include both long-acting and short-acting preparations used for relaxation of smooth muscles and bronchodilation, reducing edema, and aiding clearance of mucus. Medications include salmeterol (Serevent), sustained-release albuterol (Volmax ER®) and short-acting albuterol (Proventil), and levalbuterol (Xopenex).
- **Anticholinergics** aid in preventing bronchial constriction and potentiate the bronchodilating action of β-Adrenergic agonists. The most commonly used medication is ipratropium bromide (Atrovent).
- **Corticosteroids** provide anti-inflammatory action by inhibiting immune responses and decreasing edema, mucus, and hyper-responsiveness. Because of numerous side effects, glucocorticosteroids are usually administered orally or parenterally for ≤5 days (prednisone, prednisolone, methylprednisolone) and then switched to inhaled steroids. If a person receives glucocorticoids for more than 5 days, then dosages are tapered. Methylprednisolone IV is the standard dose for respiratory failure. The Global Initiative for Asthma (GINA) recommends daily inhaled corticosteroids for all individuals with severe asthma to reduce the risk of exacerbations.

- **Methylxanthines** are used to improve pulmonary function and decrease the need for mechanical ventilation. Medications include aminophylline and theophylline.
- **Magnesium sulfate** is used to relax smooth muscles and decrease inflammation. If administered intravenously, it must be given slowly to prevent hypotension and bradycardia. When inhaled, it potentiates the action of albuterol.
- **Heliox** (helium-oxygen) is administered to decrease airway resistance with airway obstruction, thereby decreasing respiratory effort. Heliox improves oxygenation of those on mechanical ventilation.
- **Leukotriene inhibitors** are used to inhibit inflammation and bronchospasm for long-term management. Medications include montelukast (Singulair).

ANTIHISTAMINES AND MAST CELL STABILIZERS FOR ALLERGY-RELATED ISSUES

Many respiratory problems result from the allergic response to medications and environmental allergens. The following medications are used to control this allergic response:

- **Antihistamines** work by competing for histamine binding sites, thus diminishing inflammation and bronchoconstriction. Some common antihistamines are chlorpheniramine maleate, diphenhydramine, and cetirizine.
- **Mast cell stabilizers** are used for more long-term control of asthma and other allergic diseases. Their mechanism of action is blocking histamine release from mast cells. Cromolyn is the best-known example.

SURGICAL PULMONARY INTERVENTIONS

Respiratory abnormalities may require surgery. The most common surgical thoracic procedures include the following:

- **Pneumonectomy**: Removal of a whole lung with or without resection of mediastinal lymph nodes.
- **Lobotomy**: Resection of one or more lung lobes.
- **Segmentectomy**: Excision of a section of a lung.
- **Wedge resection**: Excision of a small wedge-shaped section of lung tissue regardless of segment divisions.
- **Bronchoplasty (sleeve resection)**: Partial surgical removal and reanastomosis (reconnection) of a bronchus.
- **Laryngectomy**: Partial or complete excision of one or more vocal cords.
- **Tracheostomy**: Surgical procedure in the trachea to create a stoma or surgical opening for a tracheostomy tube.
- **Tracheal resection and reconstruction**: Partial surgical removal and reanastomosis of the trachea and/or main stem bronchi.
- **Lung volume resection**: Removal of portions of emphysematous lung tissue.
- **Rib resection**: Removal of part of one or more ribs.

NON-SURGICAL PULMONARY INTERVENTIONS

Respiratory abnormalities can also be addressed with the following non-surgical thoracic procedures:

- **Laryngoscopy**: The use of a fiberoptic scope to visualize the larynx.
- **Mediastinoscopy**: The use of an endoscope to visualize the mediastinum.
- **Pleurodesis**: The obliteration of the pleural space by introduction of a chemical agent into it using a thoracoscope (endoscope) or a thoracostomy (incision and chest tube).

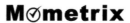

- **Thoracentesis**: The removal of pleural fluid using percutaneous needle aspiration.
- **Thoracoscopy**: Video-assisted examination of the pleura or lung tissue through the chest wall with an endoscope called a thoracoscope.

Pulmonary Physical Therapy Interventions

OUTPATIENT PULMONARY REHABILITATION
BASIC ELEMENTS

Outpatient pulmonary rehabilitation programs aim to help patients manage pulmonary disease and prepare for or recover from surgical interventions related to the pulmonary system. Patients begin outpatient pulmonary rehab once they are medically stable and cleared to do so by a medical professional. A multidisciplinary healthcare team is utilized to plan and implement rehabilitation. Programs typically include education about conditions and expectations regarding outcomes, an exercise program to improve lung function, strength training to facilitate safe completion of activities of daily living, discussions regarding healthy lifestyle changes, and stress management strategies to help maintain positive mental health. Patients are educated regarding safe use of supplemental oxygen as applicable. Providers will help strategize a return-to-work initiative with patients and employers as needed. Ultimately, patients leave pulmonary rehab with a reasonable approach to a prolonged lifespan and a favorable quality of life.

GOALS

The intent of outpatient pulmonary rehabilitation is to educate patients about lifestyle modifications that influence their condition, develop an exercise program to improve pulmonary function and increase strength, improve a patient's functional capacity for daily activities, make plans to return to work as appropriate, and develop stress management strategies. Educating patients about lifestyle factors such as nutrition, sleep hygiene, and smoking cessation provide the patient with tools to help manage their condition and reduce the risk of future pulmonary complications. Improving pulmonary function and strength enables individuals to have the capacity to safely perform activities of daily living and work tasks. Stress management strategies create a means by which patients are able to manage their mental health while dealing with potentially long-term limitations of their pulmonary disease. Medical evaluations are utilized throughout the process to document progress toward these goals and make adjustments to the plan of care when required.

EXERCISES

Outpatient pulmonary rehabilitation programs include exercise programs that incorporate aerobic activity, strength training, and specific breathing exercises. Breathing exercises can help patients stay calm and control their breath if they're feeling short of breath during daily activities. Aerobic exercise commonly includes walking, jogging, riding a bicycle, or rowing. The goals of aerobic exercises are to improve pulmonary function and impart psychological benefits. Strength training usually focuses on upper and lower body strength and may include the use of bands, ankle weights, dumbbells, barbells, or weight machines. Examples of upper body strength exercises include overhead press, lateral raises, front raises, and rows. Examples of lower body strength exercises include sit-to-stands, marching, knee extensions, hamstring curls, and box lifts. Vital signs such as blood pressure and heart rate, as well as rating of perceived exertion are objective and subjective metrics that are used during sessions to monitor the patient's response to exercise programming.

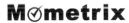

DEAN'S HIERARCHY

Dean's hierarchy for treatment of patients with impaired oxygen transport addresses bronchopulmonary hygiene. It is based on the assertion that individuals have optimal physiologic function when they are upright and moving. There are nine components:

Component	Goal	Intervention
Mobilization and exercise	To reach an exercise level that impacts the oxygen transport pathway.	Techniques ideally should result in acute, long-term, and preventive effects.
Body positioning	To position the patient as close to upright and moving as possible, whether active, assisted, or passive.	Specific positioning should impact hemodynamics due to fluid shifts and improve many cardiopulmonary functions, such as ventilation, perfusion, matching, and gas exchange.
Breathing control measures	To promote alveolar ventilation, mucociliary transport, and coughing.	Specific maneuvers of value include coordination of breathing during activity, incentive spirometry, pursed-lip breathing, eucapnic breathing, sustained maximal inspiration, and maximal tidal breaths.
Coughing maneuvers	To encourage mucociliary clearance with few cardiopulmonary side effects.	Maneuvers of value include active and spontaneous coughing with closed glottis, modified techniques with open glottis (such as a forced expiration or huffing) and active-assisted coughing.

COMPONENTS OF DEAN'S HIERARCHY

Component	Goal	Intervention
Relaxation and energy-conservation intercessions	To lessen the work of breathing, reduce unnecessary oxygen demand, and minimize heart rate.	Use of relaxation procedures while resting and active may produce energy conservation and pain control.
Range-of-motion (ROM) exercises	To stimulate alveolar ventilation and change its distribution.	Work may be active, assisted-active, or passive.
Postural drainage positioning	To assist airway clearance using gravity.	The use of bronchopulmonary segmental drainage positions.
Manual techniques	To facilitate airway clearance in combination with specific body positioning.	Procedures of value include autogenic drainage, manual percussion, vibration, use of deep breathing, and coughing.
Suctioning	To remove airway secretions.	Systems include open suction, closed suction, tracheal tickle, instillation with saline, and bagging.

BRONCHOPULMONARY HYGIENE

To institute a bronchopulmonary hygiene program for patients with respiratory issues, physical therapists and their assistants need a basic understanding of the underlying pathophysiology. They must understand concepts, such as reversibility versus irreversibility and obstructive versus restrictive lung disorders. They must also be familiar with a wide range of modalities for bronchopulmonary hygiene and know which ones require prior physician approval, such as bronchodilators, other drugs, and supplemental oxygen. Physical therapists and their assistants must be flexible in planning as physical therapy and other interventions can affect patient status. To maximize continuity, they should familiarize themselves with each patient's normal bronchopulmonary hygiene pattern. Some baseline and/or monitoring measurements are generally recommended, including baseline sputum production and pulse oximetry monitoring. Physical therapists and their assistants should be familiar with procedures to increase a patient's cough effectiveness, such as splinting, positioning, and nasotracheal suctioning of secretions.

ACTIVITY PROGRESSION IN PATIENTS WITH RESPIRATORY IMPAIRMENTS

Patients with respiratory impairments should be monitored with measurements related to respiratory function, such as the Dyspnea scale, the rating of perceived exertion, and O_2 saturation rather than heart rate. Activity progression programs should concentrate on short, frequent sessions at times when the patient will not be fatigued. Bronchopulmonary hygiene prior to the session often increases activity tolerance. The patient may need supplemental oxygen during exercise, even if not required at rest. Progression or regression should be documented, including items like type, frequency, and duration of rest periods.

PREVENTING AND ALLEVIATING DYSPNEA

Dyspnea, or shortness of breath upon exertion or exposure to allergens, commonly occurs in patients with chronic obstructive pulmonary disease (COPD). Episodes of dyspnea can be averted through a combination of controlled breathing techniques, pacing of functional activities within the individual's ventilatory capacity, and awareness. The pursed-lip breathing technique is generally used to relieve episodes of dyspnea that do occur. **Pursed-lip breathing** is believed to maintain airway patency by creating back pressure in the airways. The technique for recovery involves having patients sit or stand and bend forward, supporting themselves on a table, in order to encourage diaphragmatic breathing. They then use pursed-lip breathing during expiration, which involves breathing in slowly through the nose and then out gently through pursed or lightly touching lips. Patients should be relaxed, and they should use diaphragmatic breathing, shunning use of accessory abdominal muscles. Patients should be directed to continue this breathing until they are no longer short of breath.

PHYSICAL THERAPY FOR RESPIRATORY DYSFUNCTION

If, upon inspection, the clinician finds a patient has dyspnea, tachypnea, an asymmetric respiratory pattern, or posture issues, a number of physical therapy interventions are suggested. These include repositioning of the patient, postural exercises, relaxation techniques, energy-conservation maneuvers, trunk and shoulder stretching, incentive spirometry, and supplemental oxygen. Findings on palpation of asymmetric respiration or palpable fremitus due to pulmonary secretions suggest a range of possible interventions, including coughing maneuvers, upper-extremity and diaphragmatic exercises, postural drainage, manual techniques, functional activity, incentive spirometry, and perhaps a flutter valve. The same type of measures is indicated if there is increased dullness on percussion or decreased or unusually-positioned breath sounds on auscultation, both of which indicate retained pulmonary secretions. If the patient has an ineffective cough, possible interventions include repositioning, huffing, and coughing techniques; functional activity; a tracheal tickle (external stimulation); suctioning; bronchodilator use; and possibly incisional splinting.

POSTURAL DRAINAGE

Postural or bronchial drainage is the mobilization of secretions in lung segments from small to larger airways to be cleared by coughing or endotracheal suctioning. Patients are placed in various positions that use gravity to aid the clearing, and one or more manual techniques are used. Postural drainage is used to prevent the accumulation of secretions in those at risk for pulmonary problems, such as patients with cystic fibrosis or chronic bronchitis, those on lengthy bed rest or ventilation, or postoperative patients whose deep breathing is restricted. It is also used to remove accrued secretions from the lungs in patients with lung diseases (COPD, pneumonia, etc.), those with artificial airways, or anyone very weak. Postural drainage is contraindicated in patients who are coughing up blood, have acute untreated conditions like pulmonary edema or heart failure, are cardiovascularly unstable, or have undergone recent neurosurgery.

MANUAL TECHNIQUES

The manual techniques used for postural drainage include percussion, vibration. and shaking.

- The most common is **percussion**, where the therapist mechanically displaces thick or adherent mucus by striking the patient's chest wall rhythmically with cupped hands (or mechanically). Percussion should not be done over local fractures or tumors, nor if the individual has a pulmonary embolus, unstable angina, chest wall pain, or parameters that put them at risk for hemorrhage.
- **Vibration** is a gentle compression in the direction of chest movement and pulsation with both hands over the chest during expiration only.
- **Shaking**, which is also employed only during expiration, is a more dynamic, bouncy type of vibration in which the therapist locks their thumbs and uses both hands, directly enfolding them around the chest wall.

POSTURAL DRAINING POSITIONS FOR CLEARING THE UPPER AND MIDDLE LOBES

The seven postural drainage positions for clearing the right and left upper and middle lobes, named according to the area of clearance, are as follows:

- **Anterior apical segments**: The patient is seated using a back pillow to recline slightly back; percussion is applied under the clavicle.
- **Posterior apical segments**: The patient is seated resting forward inclined with the head on a pillow on the table; percussion is employed above the scapulae with fingers curving over the top of the shoulders.
- **Anterior segments**: The patient is supine (head up) on the table with pillows supporting the head, neck, and under the knees; percussion is employed bilaterally over the nipple or just above the breast.
- **Left posterior segment**: The patient is lying on the right side, head upward, on a table inclined 30-45° above horizontal, with a pillow under the head; percussion is employed directly over the left scapula.
- **Right posterior segment**: The patient lies flat on a table (no incline) on the left side, propped by pillows under the head and in front; percussion is applied directly over the right scapula.
- **Lingual** (projection of left upper lobe analogous to right middle lobe): The patient is lying on the right side with their head downward on a table inclined 15-30°, supported by pillows; percussion is done just under the left breast.
- **Middle lobe**: This position is similar to the lingual except the patient is lying on the left side; percussion is done under the right breast.

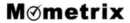

POSTURAL DRAINING POSITIONS FOR CLEARING THE LOWER LOBES

The five postural drainage positions for clearing the right and left lower lung lobes are as follows:

- **Anterior segments**: The patient lies supine on a 30-45° incline with head downward and pillow support under the knees and head; percussion is employed bilaterally over the lower portion of the ribs.
- **Posterior segments**: The patient lays prone, face on the table, and facing downward on a 30-45° incline with pillow support under the hips; percussion is done bilaterally over the lower part of the ribs.
- **Left lateral segment**: The patient lays on the right side facing downward on a 30-45° incline with pillow support; percussion is employed over the lower lateral aspect of the left rib cage.
- **Right lateral segment**: This position is similar to the left lateral segment except the patient is lying on the left side; percussion is applied over the lower lateral portion of the right rib cage.
- **Superior segments**: The patient lies prone (head down) on a non-inclined table with a pillow under the abdomen; percussion is done bilaterally, directly below the scapulae (shoulder blade).

GUIDELINES

Postural drainage is done up to four times daily depending on secretion viscosity. It is best performed before or after aerosol therapy for maximum clearance. Good times to do postural drainage are early in the morning to clear up overnight accumulation and early evening to facilitate sleeping, but never right after a meal. Sessions should last no longer than an hour as they are fatiguing. Beforehand, the patient should be taught deep breathing and effective coughing. Their clothing should be loose and thin. All needed adjunct equipment should be readily available. Establish which segments need to be drained, and check vital signs, breath sounds, and patient color before beginning. Percussion of each segment is done for 5-10 minutes with the patient breathing deeply but not hyperventilating. The patient should be persuaded to take deep double coughs as needed. If they cannot cough instinctively, they should be told to take a number of deep, successive breaths while the therapist applies vibration during expiration. The therapist moves on to the next segment as above regardless of whether there is a productive cough. Afterwards, the patient should sit up and rest while the clinician watches for indications of postural hypotension, checks vital signs and breath sounds, and characterizes secretions produced.

DIAPHRAGMATIC BREATHING

Diaphragmatic breathing is controlled breathing that maximizes utilization of the diaphragm and reduces the use of accessory muscles (shoulder, neck). This is intended to improve the efficiency of ventilation, make breathing less taxing, increase diaphragmatic movement, augment gas exchange and oxygenation, and facilitate mobilization of secretions during postural drainage. The patient should be in a position that takes advantage of gravity, such as the semi-Fowler's position. If the person instinctively employs accessory muscles, relaxation exercises, such as shoulder rolls or shrugs, should be done first. The therapist places their hand(s) on the patient's rectus abdominis below the anterior costal margin and instructs the patient to breathe in gradually and deeply through the nose and then exhale slowly via the mouth. Shoulders and upper chest should be relaxed, and the individual should refrain from hyperventilation. If necessary, inspiration can be aided by sequential nasal sniffing actions. The patient's understanding of the process can be facilitated by replacing the therapist's hand with their own to feel the movement.

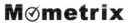

SEGMENTAL BREATHING

Segmental breathing is the expansion of localized regions of the lungs while keeping other areas quiet. It is useful for expansion of specific areas that are hypoventilated or during postural drainage procedures. One type of segmental breathing is lateral costal (lateral basal) expansion, deep breathing while concentrating on lower rib cage movement, which assists diaphragmatic excursion. This is performed first with the patient supine with legs propped, again with the patient seated, and a final time to teach the patient. The method has several steps. The therapist places their hands on the lateral aspect of the lower ribs and directs the patient to breathe out, during which the clinician applies pressure onto the patient's ribs with the palms. A rapid, downward, inward stretch is then applied. As the patient breathes in, the therapist applies gentle manual resistance to the lower ribs. The patient can use their hands, a towel, or a belt to facilitate the maneuver on their own. Another version is posterior basal expansion, recommended for patients confined to bed after surgery. The patient sits up and bends forward over a pillow. The therapist positions their hands over the posterior aspect of the lower ribs and uses the same type of pressure, stretch, and resistance sequence as for the lateral version.

POSITIVE EXPIRATORY PRESSURE AND GLOSSOPHARYNGEAL BREATHING

Positive expiratory pressure breathing uses a special mouthpiece or mask to control the resistance to airflow, thus increasing patency during exhalation and mobilizing and improving clearance of secretions. The patient is upright, if possible, in a seated position with elbows placed on a table. While wearing the mask or mouthpiece, the patient inhales, sustains the inspiration for 2-3 seconds, and exhales aided by active, but not forceful, help from the low (or sometimes higher) pressure of the device. This cycle is repeated 10-15 times, after which the patient takes off the device and coughs to discharge secretions. The sequence is reiterated several more times, up to about 15 minutes in total.

Glossopharyngeal breathing is used primarily in patients who require mechanical ventilation due to some sort of neuromuscular damage that influences the innervation of the diaphragm. The main purpose of the technique is to enhance inspiratory capacity. The patient takes a series of up to about 10 gulps of air and then closes the mouth. They then use the tongue to move air back and trap it in the pharynx. When the glottis opens, the air is propelled into the lungs.

RESPIRATORY RESISTANCE TRAINING

Respiratory resistance training (RRT) is a strengthening of or improvement in the endurance of ventilatory muscles in patients with pulmonary diseases that have damaged these muscles. Most RRT concentrates on training the muscles of inspiration, such as the abdominal muscles and diaphragm. The major types of RRT are:

- **Inspiratory resistance training**: This is designed to strengthen and improve the stamina of the muscles of inspiration by making them work harder. The patient breathes in through the mouth via a resistive training apparatus (pressure or airflow-based) for an indicated amount of time several times daily. The time of use is increased periodically up to 20-30 minutes per session.
- **Incentive respiratory spirometry**: This is designed to increase the volume of air inspired. It is generally used post-surgically to avert alveolar collapse and atelectasis. The patient is placed in a semi-reclined or other comfortable position and asked to breath normally four times with maximum expiration on the fourth breath. They then put a spirometer (a small device that provides feedback on whether maximum inspiration is achieved) in the mouth and inhale maximally for several seconds through its mouthpiece to a goal setting. This is done 5-10 times daily.

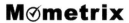

EXERCISES TO MOBILIZE THE CHEST

Chest mobilization exercises are any drills that mix active movements of the trunk with deep breathing. These exercises are indicated when the lack of mobility of trunk muscles impacts ventilation or postural alignment. Some specific exercises include:

- **Mobilization of one side of the chest**: The seated patient bends away from the taut side for lengthening and chest expansion. They then use a fisted hand to push into the tight lateral aspect while bending into that tight side and exhaling. They can also lift the arm on the taut side and bend to the opposite side for further stretch.
- **Mobilization of the upper chest and stretching of pectoralis muscles**: The patient is seated in a chair with hands clutched behind the head. They pull the arms back during deep inspiration and forward until elbows touch during expiration.
- **Mobilization of the upper chest and shoulders**: While seated, the individual lifts both arms directly overhead during inspiration and then bends fully forward, touching the floor during expiration.

COUGH MECHANISM

Normally, the cough pump, or cough mechanism, follows a series of steps. In order to cough, a person takes a deep inspiration, after which the glottis closes and the vocal cords tighten. The abdominal muscles contract and the diaphragm rises up, a combination that increases intrathoracic and intraabdominal pressures. Next, the glottis opens, and air is expelled, or expired. Cilia in the epithelial layers of the bronchial tree normally help facilitate the expulsion of secretions.

The cough mechanism is compromised if there is decreased inspiratory capacity due to factors like lung disease, chest trauma, thoracic or abdominal surgery, or injuries that impact neuromuscular control (such as spinal cord injury). Spinal cord injuries above the T12 level or other muscular diseases, such as muscular dystrophy, weaken abdominals, making it difficult to forcibly expel air. Procedures such as intubation and anesthesia, as well as some lung diseases, diminish ciliary action. Similarly, certain procedures (e.g., intubation) and certain conditions (for example, cystic fibrosis) increase or thicken mucus production.

TEACHING A PATIENT TO PERFORM AN EFFECTIVE COUGH

After observing the patient's cough, have them assume a relaxed position, preferably seated or leaning forward slightly. The patient is taught controlled diaphragmatic breathing using deep inspirations. The therapist then demonstrates a deep double cough, as well as the correct muscle action of abdominal contraction during coughing. Patients should experience this contraction by placing their hands on their own abdomen and huffing three times upon expiration. Another way to feel a contraction is to make a "K" sound. The patient is then told to take, in sequence, a deep inspiration and a sharp double cough. An effective cough is generally observed after two rounds. Patients with weak inspiratory or abdominal muscles may need an abdominal binder or they may need to use glossopharyngeal breathing. Patients should never be permitted to gasp in air since this can cause fatigue, increased airway resistance, and/or mucus plugging.

ADJUNCT TECHNIQUES FOR EFFECTIVE COUGHING AND AIRWAY CLEARANCE

There are manual-assisted methods (both therapist and self types) to improve coughing and airway clearance. Manual-assisted cough techniques enhance the cough mechanism by applying pressure to the abdominal area, which creates more intra-abdominal pressure and forceful coughing. For therapist-assisted manual cough techniques, the patient is either supine (or semi-reclined) or seated. In the supine method, the therapist places the heels of both hands, one on top of the other, on the patient's abdomen just distal to the xiphoid process (lowest segment of breastbone). The

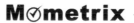

therapist manually aids the patient during the coughing and expiration phase by compressing the abdomen inward and upward, thrusting the diaphragm upward. If the patient is seated, the therapist stands behind the patient and applies similar pressure. In the self-assisted technique, the patient is seated with arms crossed over the abdomen or intertwined hands below the xiphoid process. They should use the wrists or forearms to do the same type of pushing while leaning forward during the coughing phase. Self-assistance may also include splinting (use of pillow or hands over an incision during coughing), humidification, and/or tracheal stimulation.

MANAGEMENT OF POST-THORACIC SURGERY PATIENTS

Patients who have undergone thoracic surgery have substantial chest pain, which makes lung expansion, chest wall mobility, and coughing difficult. Thus, they are prone to accretion of pulmonary secretions and secondary issues, such as pneumonia. In addition, the general anesthesia used during the procedure depresses ciliary action, cough reflexes, and the respiratory center, while the intubation procedure further decreases ciliary action, irritates the mucosal surfaces, and initiates muscle spasms. Pain at the incision depresses chest wall compliance and effective coughing, resulting in shallow breathing and cough. Pain medications given postoperatively also tend to depress the respiratory center and ciliary activity. Post-surgery, the patient is weak and sedentary, leading to pooling of secretions and inefficiency of the cough pump. All of these factors make it essential that a comprehensive program incorporates breathing and coughing exercises, secretion removal, shoulder range-of-motion exercises, posture awareness instruction, and graded aerobic conditioning.

CARE PLAN

The patient's status is first determined in terms of vital signs, sputum drainage into chest tubes, etc. The individual should be placed in a semi-Fowler's position, an approximate 30° elevation of the bed's head, coupled with slight flexion in the knees and hips, to support relaxation and reduce pain by placing less traction on the incision. Steps to optimize ventilation and re-inflate lung tissue should be initiated to prevent pneumonia or collapsed lung. Deep breathing exercises are initiated on the day of surgery (continuing until the patient is ambulatory), followed by the addition of incentive spirometry or inspiratory resistance exercises. Once the patient is alert, measures to support secretion removal should be instituted, including effective coughing, functional mobility, and modified postural drainage if secretions accrue. Lower-extremity exercises, such as ankle pumping, should be started a day post-surgery to optimize circulation there and prevent DVT and PE. To recoup range of motion (ROM) in the shoulders, shoulder relaxation, active-assistive, and, eventually, active ROM exercises should be initiated. Correct postural alignment (symmetrical) and trunk positioning should be taught. Once chest tubes are eliminated and the patient can get up, progressive graded ambulation or stationary cycling should be started to increase exercise tolerance.

Musculoskeletal System

Physical Therapy Data Collection

STRUCTURE AND FUNCTION OF THE MUSCULOSKELETAL SYSTEM

The musculoskeletal system is comprised of the bony skeleton and soft tissues. The soft tissues include contractile muscles, tough fibrous tendons and ligaments, joint capsules, and relatively elastic cartilage. The musculoskeletal system enables movement and performance of fine-motor tasks, absorbs shock, converts and generates energy, and protects vital organs and the central nervous system. The musculoskeletal system is intimately related to the nervous system as nerves stimulate the muscles. Functional deficits are often related to impairment of the musculoskeletal system through traumatic injuries or degenerative alterations.

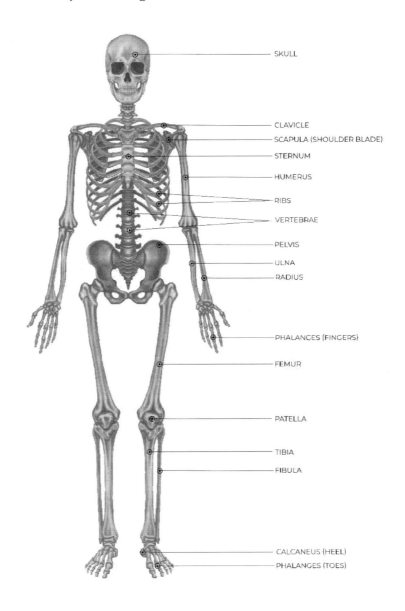

84

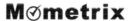

JOINT ABNORMALITIES IN RELATION TO MUSCULOSKELETAL ISSUES

Joints must perform properly for movement and range of motion. Joints that are **locking** cannot be completely extended and generally cannot go through a full range of motion. **Pseudolocking** is similar but refers to a lack of extension and flexion at different times. **Spasm** locking occurs with muscle spasm or quick movement. Another joint problem is **giving way** due to weak muscles or inhibition of reflexes. **Joint laxity** is greater than normal range of motion, which can generally be controlled and is not pathological; it is related to ligament function and joint capsule resistance. Joint laxity that is associated with symptoms and pathology and cannot be controlled is called hypermobility. **Hypermobility** results in various types of joint instability.

TYPES OF JOINT INSTABILITY

Joint instability is excessive, uncontrollable, pathologically derived joint hypermobility. For observational purposes, there are two general types of joint instability.

- The first is **translational instability**, the loss of small, arthrokinematic joint movements.
- The other is **anatomical instability**, which is more excessive and precedent to dislocation or subluxation (partial dislocation).

Both types can cause functional instability, or the lack of ability to control joint movement during functional activities. Both can also be initiated voluntarily through muscle contraction or involuntarily due to positioning. When assessing joint stability, the observer should look for injuries on both sides of the joint (the circle concept of instability).

PATIENT HISTORY

In addition to general medical questions, there are specific areas related to possible musculoskeletal problems that should be addressed in the patient history. The examiner should ask about the individual's chief complaint or history of the present illness, the mechanism of injury, the rapidity of onset of symptoms, areas that bother the patient, types of sensations and their locations, and particularly the history and characterization of the involved pain. Mechanism of injury refers to whether there was a provoking trauma (macrotrauma) or a repetitive activity (microtrauma) involved. Previous history of musculoskeletal, rheumatologic, or neurologic diseases should be noted along with prior injuries and surgeries, use of assistive devices or adaptive equipment, and history of falls. The history should also include potentially relevant information, such as the use of analgesics, steroids, or other medications; physician precautions regarding weight bearing, activity level, or positioning; lab and imaging information; and familial or developmental history of diseases, such as cancer or arthritis and other serious systemic illnesses.

DATA COLLECTION
OBSERVATIONS

The three most important things to observe when assessing the musculoskeletal system are the patient's posture, limb position, and skin integrity. Normal standing posture and gait should be observed surreptitiously before the formal data collection process. Indications of overt pain include guarding (stiff, rigid movements), bracing weight primarily on one extended limb, rubbing the painful area, grimacing, and sighing accompanied by movement. The formal data collection process is performed in a private area with the patient in underwear. Here, the observer should note whether the patient's body alignment is straight and whether there are any noticeable structural or functional deformities that restrict range of motion, cause malalignment, change bone shape, or cause dislocation. The patient's resting posture should be observed standing, sitting, and supine, including observation of head, neck, and extremities for alignment, symmetry, atrophy, and deformities. The limb positions should be observed for equality and symmetry, including factors

85

like size, color, position, temperature, etc. The skin should be inspected for integrity, scarring, color changes, bruising, texture, lacerations, edema, pressure sores, and surgical incisions. The examiner should also note crepitus, snapping, or other abnormal sounds in joints during movement.

OBSERVATION OF ACTIVE MOVEMENTS

Stated in order, active, passive, and resisted isometric movements are tested during examination for potential musculoskeletal problems. Patients should be asked to perform active or physiological movements, unless a fracture is healing or stress would be put on recently healed soft tissues. The examiner observes and records the point at which pain occurs, whether the movement intensifies the pain, the quality of the pain, the patient's reaction, the extent and nature of restriction, the movement pattern and rhythm, and the movement of associated joints. It is important to note whether the patient uses cheating or trick movements to complete the activity, such as shoulder hiking, and where in the arc of movement the symptoms transpire.

OBSERVATION OF PASSIVE MOVEMENTS

Passive, or anatomical, movements are generally observed after active movements. Passive movements involve putting the joint through gentle movements within its range of motion (ROM) while the patient is relaxed. Just as with active movements, the examiner should note when and where during each movement pain is initiated, if the movement increases the intensity and quality of pain, limitations to movement, and movement of associated joints. Measurements of the angles for range of motion are estimated or, preferably quantified, with instruments such as a goniometer or inclinometer. The normal expected joint mobility varies for individuals, but in general, if outside the functional range, it can be classified as limited hypomobility or excessive hypermobility (laxity). Another important observation is the end feel, which is the sensation the examiner feels by applying overpressure at the end of the ROM.

PALPATION

Palpation with finger pressure to detect tenderness should be done after identification of the affected tissue. The unaffected side is palpated first, and the palpation is done in a systematic manner. The supported body part is felt for differences in tissue tension, muscle tone, tissue texture, tissue thickness, joint tenderness, temperature disparities, pulses, tremors, fasciculations (inflamed connective tissues), the pathological state of the joint or surrounding tissues, dryness or excess moisture, and any abnormal sensations. According to the pain pressure threshold (PPT) scale supported by the APTA, tenderness is graded according to patient complaints as I (pain only), II (pain and wincing), III (wincing and withdrawing of the joint), or IV (palpation not permitted by patient). In particular, tissue thickness can indicate swelling (the abnormal enlargement of a body part due to bone or synovial membrane thickening) or fluid accumulation (edema) in or near the joint. Characteristic feelings of swelling on palpation are acute, hard, warm, tense swelling, suggesting blood accumulation; a boggy, spongy feeling, appearing 8-24 hours after occurrence and indicating inflammation and synovial swelling; hard, implying bone swelling; thick and slow-moving with pitting edema; etc.

NORMAL END FEEL

End feel is the sensation the examiner feels while applying overpressure at the end of a range-of-motion test (passive or, sometimes, active). It is a subjective parameter, but with time should become consistent for the particular examiner. The Cyriax classification system is often used. This system identifies three normal end feels:

- **Bone to bone**: Hard and painless, such as with elbow extension.
- **Soft tissue approximation**: A spongy compressive feel, such as with elbow or knee flexion.

86

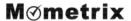

- **Tissue stretch**: Either elastic (soft) or capsular (hard), depending on the thickness and type of tissue being stretched; due to capsule or ligament issues, such as shoulder lateral rotation or ankle dorsiflexion.

ABNORMAL END FEELS

There are many possible abnormal end feels during examination for range of motion (ROM) that are good diagnostic aids for pinpointing the associated problem. Muscle spasms, or movement followed by abrupt halting, can occur early or late in the ROM. Early muscle spasms are generally due to acute injury and inflammation, whereas late muscle spasms are primarily a result of instability. Spasticity, due to upper motor neuron lesions, may feel fairly similar. Tight muscles have a sensation similar to normal tissue stretch but 'mushier.' An abnormal bone-to-bone end feel is one in which the constraint occurs before the normal end of ROM or at an unusual time, usually due to bony growths. Reduced ROM from capsular issues can give a hard capsular end feel, similar to tissue stretch but thicker, or a soft capsular end feel, which is akin to normal tissue stretch but with restricted ROM. Examples of abnormal hard or soft capsular responses include frozen shoulders and synovial inflammation, respectively. Other abnormal types are an empty end feel, which is very painful and indicates no mechanical resistance, such as with acute subacromial bursitis; and springy block type, a tissue stretch in an unexpected place, usually a joint with a meniscus, such as a knee meniscus tear.

PATTERNS OF LIMITATION

Capsular patterns of limitation, or restriction, are observed when joints controlled by muscles are involved. The possible causes are muscle spasms, capsular contractions, and osteophyte (bony growth) formation. The list of common capsular patterns of joints is extensive, with examples including restricted mouth opening for the temporomandibular joint, limitations of the hip joint (flexion, abduction, medial rotation), restricted knee flexion or extension, side flexion, rotation and extension for the thoracic or lumbar spine, and many others.

Atypical patterns are considered **noncapsular patterns of limitation**, which may be due to an absent capsular reaction, ligamentous adhesion, internal derangement (at knee, ankle, or elbow), or extra-articular lesion, which influences the joint restricted.

EVALUATING FOR INERT TISSUE PROBLEMS

Inert tissues are those that are not contractile (muscles, tendons, attachments) or nervous tissues. Inert tissues include ligaments, joint capsules, bursae (fluid-filled sacs), cartilage, blood vessels, and dura mater (nervous tissue covering). Evaluations for inert tissue problems should be done after active and passive movements. If there are lesions in inert tissues, one of four typical patterns for range-of-motion (ROM) restriction will be observed:

- **Painless, full ROM**: Suggesting no lesion on the inert tissues being tested
- **Pain and limited ROM in every direction**: Indicative of total joint involvement, as seen with arthritis or capsulitis
- **Pain with limited or excessive ROM in some directions but not others**: Caused by anything that produces a noncapsular pattern of limitation
- **Painless, limited ROM**: Typically due to osteoarthritis

RESISTED ISOMETRIC MOVEMENTS FOR EVALUATING THE JOINTS

Resisted isometric movements are strong voluntary muscle contractions done with the joint in a resting position. The joint angle and muscle length are kept constant. Characteristic isometric movements involve holding something or pressing against an immovable force. They are performed after other testing. They test primarily for pain elicited in contractile tissues (muscle, tendon), the bone insertion, or associated innervation because extraneous movement that might involve inert tissues is minimized. Isometric movements are appropriate only with a muscle strength grade between 3 and 5, which is basically some-to-complete range of motion against gravity. The examiner observes the strength of the contraction and whether the contraction causes pain. If pain was caused, the intensity and quality of pain should be noted, in addition to the type of contraction triggering the problem. This may require adjunct methods, such as testing for eccentric or concentric contractions. Resisted isometric movements should cause pain in the same direction as active movements if there is some type of contractile (muscle strain, tendinopathies) or associated (nervous system, avulsion, psychological) weakness.

PAIN AND MOVEMENT PATTERNS

Resisted isometric movements mainly test for pain associated with contractile and nervous system tissues. There are four typical patterns seen:

- **Painless, strong movement**: Indicates noninvolvement of the area being tested; can be due to first- or second-degree muscle strains, which cause reflex inhibition and weakness or cogwheel contractions
- **Pain and relatively strong movement**: Implies some sort of local muscle or tendon lesion; can also be caused by avulsion fractures or tendinopathies, including tendinosis (intratendinous degeneration), peritenonitis (inflammation of the external layer of the tendon), a combination of the two, or tendonitis/partial rupture of the tendon
- **Pain and weak movement**: Indicates a fracture or other severe joint lesion
- **Painless, weak movement**: Due to contractile or nervous issues; usually caused by neurologic involvement at the peripheral nerve or nerve root level, tendon rupture, or, to a lesser extent, third-degree muscle strains (visible bulge often observed)

POSTURAL VS. PHASIC MUSCLES

The concept of postural versus phasic muscles was expounded by Janda, who maintained that muscles are either postural or phasic.

- **Postural**, or tonic, muscles are those needed to preserve upright posture, thus making them prone to tightness and hypertonicity. This includes muscles like the gastrocnemius and soleus in the calf, the erector spinae associated with the spine, the pectoralis major, hamstrings, and many others. In addition to postural functions, these muscles are associated with flexor reflexes, generally connect to two joints, are promptly activated during movement, and are resistant to atrophy.
- Most other muscles are **phasic** muscles not directly involved in postural functions, such as the rectus abdominis, external obliques, and gluteus maximus. Phasic muscles are more prone to atrophy, inhibition, hypotonia, and weakness. They are primarily one-joint muscles, generally associated with extensor reflexes, and not quickly activated during movement.

There can be both tight hypertonic postural and weak lengthened phasic muscles at a particular joint. There are generally force couples, or counteracting groups of muscles, around joints that can disrupt balance, stability, or smoothness of movement if one muscle is weak.

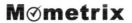

TYPES OF MUSCLE CONTRACTIONS

Types of muscle contractions include the following:

- **Eccentric contractions** are more dynamic and involve generation of a force that is less than the external load, during which muscle fibers lengthen. Eccentric contractions are sometimes used as breaks during resisted isometric movements to distinguish between grade 4 (good) and grade 5 (normal) range of motion.
- **Concentric contractions** are those in which enough force is generated to overcome a resistance and the muscle shortens during the contraction.
- An **isometric contraction** is one in which the joint angle and muscle length are kept constant, such as holding something or pressing against an immovable force.
- **Isotonic contractions** are those in which the muscle changes length but the tension is kept constant, such as those that occur when the force of contraction exceeds the load on the muscle.

FUNCTIONAL ASSESSMENT

Functional assessment is an analysis of the limitations placed on the activities the patient considers important. This is primarily performed by the physical therapist, but should be noted by the physical therapist assistant as well. It is primarily subjective and should be individualized. It evaluates the individual's ability to perform whole-body tasks, rather than move individual joints as examined by other tests. The types of functional activities that should be evaluated, if appropriate, include self-care activities (bathing, eating, going to bathroom, etc.), recreational activities, grocery shopping, work-related activities, walking, sports-related activities, etc. A good guideline is to evaluate the four areas of human function described by Goldstein:

- **Basic or personal activities of daily living (ADLs)**: Including bedtime, hygiene, eating, dressing, transfer, and walking activities.
- **Instrumental or advanced ADLs**: Such as meal preparation, shopping, light housework, check writing, communicating, driving, or sexual intercourse.
- **Work activities**: Including lifting, carrying, pulling, etc.
- **Sport and recreational activities**: Such as walking, other participatory sports, and drills for agility, reaction time, endurance, etc.

FUNCTIONAL ASSESSMENT TOOLS

There are many functional assessment tools available to the physical therapist that assistants should be aware of as well. The most important consideration with each is that they reliably and inclusively evaluate functions that are important to the patient. Questionnaires ask about daily living skills and mobility. Some use numerical scoring systems that assign different ratings to the extent of each functionality the examiner considers important, as with the Shoulder Evaluation Form, which assigns ratings to the degree of pain, stability, motion, etc., in the shoulder. Some ask the patient to rate the difficulty of performing a particular task or how much the patient is bothered by certain problems as currently perceived; an example is the Short Musculoskeletal Function Assessment (SMFA) questionnaire. Actual functional tests, such as the upper-extremity function test, timed leg standing, tandem walking, or specific activity tests, are used to simulate activities of daily living to see how well the patient can perform them and, in some cases, provoke symptoms for evaluation.

JOINT PLAY AND JOINT POSITIONS

Joint play, or accessory movement, refers to the involuntary, small range of motion (ROM) that can be achieved through passive movement by the examiner. Joint play, generally 4 mm or more in any direction, is essential for painless voluntary movement of the joint and full ROM. Therefore, joint play testing is a part of musculoskeletal evaluation. It should be done with both patient and examiner relaxed. The patient is fully supported, and one joint and one movement are evaluated at a time. The uninvolved side is tested first. One articular surface is stabilized while the other is moved. Joint play movements should be assessed with the joint in the loose-packed, or resting, position where there is least stress, not the close-packed, or synarthrodial position, which is more compressed and places joint structures under tension. However, the close-packed position offers maximal joint stability, making it ideal for stabilization of one joint while treating an adjacent one. The resting position should be used for resistive isometric movements.

RESTING AND CLOSE-PACKED POSITIONS

Each joint has a relatively non-stressed resting position and a compressed, tenser close-packed position. For the major hip and knee joints, the resting position is some flexion, while the close-packed position is full extension with rotation. The foot joints are resting when positioned midway between extremes of range of movement and close-packed when the sole is turned upward. The temporomandibular joint is relaxed with the mouth slightly open and close-packed with clenched teeth. The resting and close-packed positions of each joint are very specific to the joint, and the examiner may need to refer to specific listings for each.

GAIT
NORMAL GAIT CYCLE

The gait cycle is the time period or series of motions that transpire between two consecutive initial contacts of the same foot. The other foot has its own gait cycle, which is 180° out of phase with it. There are two phases for each foot. The **stance phase** comprises approximately 60% of the cycle and starts with the foot on the ground, bearing weight. It consists of five phases:

1. The initial contact, or heel strike
2. The load response, where the foot is flat
3. The midstance
4. The terminal stance, where the heel comes off the ground
5. The pre-swing, when the toe comes off the ground

Initial contact comprises 10% of the gait cycle and is considered a double-limb support or double-leg stance. The load response and midstance combined take up 40% of the cycle and are considered single-limb supports or single-leg stances. The combined terminal stance and pre-swing portions are approximately 10% of the gait cycle and make up the second double-limb support or weight-unloading period.

The foot then enters the **swing phase**, which comprises about 40% of the gait cycle and consists of three phases:

1. The initial swing, or acceleration forward, during which the knee and ankle flex and the limb swings.
2. The mid-swing, when the swing and other leg are side-by-side.
3. The terminal swing, or deceleration, where the leg slows in preparation for the next cycle.

FLOAT PHASE OF GAIT

When a person is running or otherwise ambulating quickly, gait cycle changes somewhat. During walking, the stance phase comprises about 60-65% of the gait cycle, with the swing phase making up the rest. During running, there are two float phases, or double unsupported phases, in between stance-swing and swing-stance, each making up about 15% of the cycle (for a total of approximately

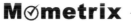

30%). This, accordingly, shortens the stance and swing phases. Joint movements are similar to those for walking but encompass a greater range of motion; for example, there is considerably more hip flexion during running, particularly in the float phases.

MUSCLE GROUPS INVOLVED IN THE PHASES OF GAIT

The muscle groups involved during gait are reflective of the mechanical goals of each portion. During the initial-contact instant of the stance phase, the goals are positioning the foot, initiation of deceleration, and use of the ankle dorsiflexors, hip extensors, and knee flexors. During the loading-response phase, the objectives are acceptance of the weight, stabilization of the pelvis, and deceleration, which uses the knee extensors, hip abductors, and ankle plantar flexors. The midstance serves to stabilize the knee, while maintaining momentum; and the goal of the terminal-stance portion is mass acceleration. Both use ankle plantar flexors but differently, namely isometrically for midstance and concentrically for terminal stance. The pre-swing serves as preparation for the swing phase and employs the hip flexors. The beginning of the swing phase, the initial swing, is used to clear the foot and change cadence, which necessitates use of the ankle dorsiflexors and hip flexors. Clearing of the foot and use of the ankle dorsiflexor continues during mid-swing. The goals of the terminal swing are deceleration of the shank and leg, positioning of the foot, and preparation for contact, utilizing knee flexors and extensors, hip extensors, and ankle dorsiflexors.

OBSERVATIONS MADE DURING THE GAIT ASSESSMENT

During observation, male patients should wear shorts, females should wear shorts and a bra, and all should usually be barefoot. The physical therapist observes the patient's posture, degree of symmetry, and general gait parameters (utilizing aids if necessary). They observe the patient's gait from the front, side, and back, each directionally, which means that for the stance phase, the direction is from the foot up to the pelvis and lumbar spine and vice versa for the swing phase. The movement pattern of the upper limbs is also noted. The salient observation points from the anterior or posterior views are undesired presence of pelvic tilt or rotation; presence of reciprocal arm swing, as desired; rotation of the trunk and upper limb in opposition to the pelvis, as expected; muscle atrophy of the thigh or leg; the positioning at various gait phases; toe angling (should be 5-18° outward); and normal behavior of hip, knee, ankle, and foot joints, as well as the tibia. The anterior and posterior views are superior for observation of the weight-loading and weight-unloading portions of gait, respectively. The lateral view is good for observation of shoulder and thorax rotation, spinal posture, joint movements, gait parameters (such as step or stride length), and coordination of movement.

OBSERVATIONS TO MAKE DURING THE INITIAL CONTACT PORTION OF THE STANCE PHASE

The stance phase of the gait cycle is considered the closed kinetic chain phase of gait because the foot is fixed and joints must adjust. If gait is normal, each instant or portion of the stance phase produces characteristic kinematic motion regardless of force. There are also typical kinetic motions, both external reaction forces and internal forces of muscles. For the initial contact or heel-strike portion of the stance phase, the expected kinematic motions are: 20-40° flexion of the hip moving toward extension, plus minor adduction and lateral rotation; the knee in full extension prior to heel contact and flexing during the heel strike; the tibia in slight lateral rotation; the foot in rigid supination (sole upward) at the point of heel contact; and the ankle moving toward plantar flexion. Abnormal responses to look for include increased knee flexion or early plantar flexion, indicating pain; tactics to extend the knee, suggesting some sort of weakness there; and touching down of other parts of the foot before heel strike, generally suggestive of some muscular or neurological issue.

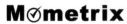

OBSERVATIONS TO MAKE DURING THE LOAD-RESPONSE PORTION OF THE STANCE PHASE

The load-response or foot flat portion of the stance phase is also called the weight acceptance instant because it is the point at which the person chooses to bear weight on the limb. Expected normal kinematic motions during the load-response portion of the stance phase are: the hip moving into extension, adduction, and medial rotation; the knee flexed approximately 20° moving toward extension; the tibia in medial rotation; the foot in pronation (rotated somewhat inward with weight born on the inside); and the ankle in plantar flexion to dorsiflexion over the fixed foot. Excessive or absent knee motion during this phase suggests weak quadriceps, plasticity, or contractures of the plantar flexor.

OBSERVATIONS TO MAKE DURING THE MIDSTANCE PORTION OF THE STANCE PHASE

During the midstance or single-leg support instant, the trunk should be above the supporting foot with evenly distributed weight and the pelvis should drop somewhat to the swing leg side. The normal expected kinematic motions at each joint are: the hip moving through a neutral position, with the pelvis rotating posteriorly; the knee flexed 15°, shifting toward extension; the tibia in medial rotation; the foot neutral; and the ankle in slight (3°) dorsiflexion. Any painful joint pathology, such as arthritis, fallen arches, or plantar fasciitis, will cause the individual to shorten this phase. Rolling off of this phase is a positive Trendelenburg's sign caused by weakness of the gluteus medius nerve root.

OBSERVATIONS TO MAKE DURING THE WEIGHT-UNLOADING PORTION OF THE STANCE PHASE

During the heel-off or terminal-stance portion of the weight-unloading period, the trunk moves toward the stance leg and the pelvis is posteriorly rotated. The normal joint kinematic movements are: a 10-15° extension of hip abduction with lateral rotation; the knee flexing 4°, moving toward extension; the tibia in lateral rotation; the foot in supination as it stiffens for push-off; and the ankle in 15° dorsiflexion toward plantar flexion. During the toe-off or pre-swing instant while acceleration is initiated, the hip is normally moving toward a 10° extension in abduction and lateral rotation; the knee moves from close to full extension to 40° flexion; the tibia is in lateral rotation; the foot is in supination; and the ankle is in 20° plantar flexion. Indications of pain during the pre-swing period suggest some sort of pathology related to the hallux (great toe), often in the metatarsophalangeal joint. Inability to push off indicates weak plantar flexors and sacral nerve root issues.

OBSERVATIONS TO MAKE DURING THE SWING PHASE

During the swing phase of the gait cycle, the involved lower extremity is said to be in an open kinetic chain because the foot is not fixed to the ground and the limb and joints are less stressed than during most of the stance phase. During the initial swing or acceleration instant of the swing phase into the mid-swing, the hip is slightly flexed (up to 15°) and medially rotated. The knee increasingly flexes up to 30-60°, with lateral rotation of the tibia moving toward neutral. The foot and ankle are in an approximate 20° dorsiflexion with some pronation. Excessive hip flexion during mid-swing indicates drop foot. Moving from mid-swing into the terminal swing or deceleration portion, the hip flexes more, to approximately 30-40°; the knee should be almost fully extended with slight lateral tibial rotation; the ankle is normally neutral; and the foot is in slight supination.

EXAMINATION PORTION OF THE GAIT ASSESSMENT

The examination portion of gait assessment consists of measurement of the parameters of gait to compare left and right gait cycles; measurement of each leg to look for differences; and often, the use of locomotion scales, grading systems, or other functional tests. These locomotion scales are often tailored to the population the patient falls into, for example, people with rheumatoid arthritis or the elderly. Gait-related parameters beyond the amount and type of joint movement are

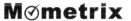

generally included, for example, the ability to climb stairs or the degree of guardedness during portions of the gait cycle. An important aspect of the examination portion is determination of whether the patient is employing compensatory mechanisms. The physical therapist will perform and document this assessment, which should then be reviewed with the assistant prior to physical therapy interventions.

NORMAL GAIT PARAMETERS

Normal parameters of gait should be observed in individuals from about 8-45 years of age. Many factors are decreased in women compared to men, in older individuals, etc. Parameters and their normal ranges are as follows:

- The **normal base width** between the two feet is 5-10 cm (2-4 inches).
- The typical step, or **gait length**, between the contact points of the two feet is approximately 72 cm or 28 inches, although this parameter is affected by many factors, including age, height, sex (less in females), etc.
- The **stride length** should be double the gait length, about 144 cm, and is the linear distance between similar points of contact on a particular foot (i.e., the gait cycle).
- **Lateral pelvic shift or list**, which is pelvic side movement during walking, should be minimal, only 2.5-5.0 cm, as should vertical pelvic shift.
- **Normal pelvic rotation** is 8° (4° each, forward on the swing leg and posteriorly on the stance leg), with the thorax moving in the other direction simultaneously.
- The **center of gravity shifts** in a figure eight pattern within a 5 cm square area, which makes the head descend or ascend during weight-loading or weight-unloading periods, respectively.
- A **customary cadence** is 90-120 steps per minute, with women usually taking 6-9 steps a minute more and older people taking fewer. An average gait speed is 1.4 meters per second or 3 mph.

ANTALGIC GAIT

Abnormal gait patterns have three sources: joint pathology or injury, compensation for these in joints on the same side of the body, or compensation on the opposite side. Antalgic gait is abnormal painful gait due to injury to the pelvis or any of the major joints from the hip down. It is seen with various forms of arthritis, osteomyelitis, tumors, foreign bodies in the foot, and various other conditions. The patient tries to take weight off the affected limb as rapidly as possible, making the stance phase for that leg relatively short, reducing the step length on the uninvolved side, and decreasing walking velocity and cadence. The individual often supports the painful area with a hand or arm and may transfer body weight over a painful hip.

GLUTEUS MAXIMUS AND GLUTEUS MEDIUS GAITS

Gluteus maximus and gluteus medius gaits are two abnormal gait patterns. Gluteus maximus gait has a distinctive backward lurch of the trunk on initial contact, which compensates for a weak gluteus maximus muscle, allowing hip extension.

Gluteus medius, or Trendelenburg's gait, is excessive lateral list toward the stance leg, compensating for weak abductor muscles in the buttocks, the gluteus medius, or the gluteus minimus. If gluteus medius muscles on both sides are weak, there is noticeable side-to-side movement. The pattern is called Trendelenburg's gait because there is a positive Trendelenburg's sign, which is drooping on the contralateral side. This gait can also be seen with congenital hip dislocation and deformities.

ARTHROGENIC AND CONTRACTURE GAITS

Arthrogenic and contracture gaits are two abnormal gait patterns generally due to previous prolonged immobilization. An arthrogenic (stiff knee or hip) gait, also caused by fusion at the joint, is a pattern whereby the individual uses plantar flexion of the opposing ankle and circumduction of the stiff extremity to lift the entire affected leg higher than usual for clearance.

In contracture gaits, the person uses compensatory mechanisms to counteract contractures for clearance. There are several patterns depending on the site of contracture. For example, increased lumbar lordosis combined with trunk extension and knee flexion is indicative of a hip flexion contraction.

ABNORMAL GAIT PATTERNS ASSOCIATED WITH CONGENITAL DEFORMITIES

One abnormal gait pattern observed primarily in patients with congenital deformities is equinus gait of toe walking. This pattern is associated with children that have congenital talipes equinovarus, or clubfoot, which is internal rotation of the foot at the ankle. These children rotate their pelvis and femur laterally for compensation, bear weight during gait on the dorsolateral or lateral portion of the foot, limp, and exhibit a shortened weight-bearing phase. Short leg, or painless estrogenic gait occurs when a person has differing leg lengths or a deformity in a leg bone. The patient shifts laterally toward the affected side, tilting the pelvis and walking with a limp. Possible additional abnormalities of gait include supination of the foot on the involved side, increased flexion in the uninvolved limb, and hiking of the hip during the swing phase.

ABNORMAL GAIT PATTERS ASSOCIATED WITH NEUROLOGIC ISSUES

Abnormal gait patterns that are generally neurologic in origin include:

- **Ataxic gait**: Seen in patients with poor sensation or lack of muscle control; characterized by poor balance, wide base, staggering or exaggerated movements, slapping of the feet, and looking downward.
- **Hemiplegic or hemiparetic gait**: Also known as neurogenic or flaccid gait; characterized by outward swinging or pushing of the paraplegic leg and use of upper limb across the trunk for balance.
- **Parkinsonian gait**: Distinguished by flexion of neck, trunk, and knees, shuffling or short steps, and absence of normal arm movement.
- **Scissors gait**: Also known as neurogenic or spastic gait; due to spastic paralysis of the hip adductors; patient draws knees together during gait.
- **Steppage or drop foot gait**: Due to loss of control of dorsiflexor muscles as a result of muscle or nerve damage; compensatory pattern in which the individual lifts the knee too high and then slaps the foot on the floor.

ABNORMAL GAIT PATTERNS ASSOCIATED WITH MUSCLE WEAKNESS

In addition to gluteus maximus and gluteus medius gaits, other common abnormal gait patterns due to muscle weakness include:

- **Quadriceps avoidance gait**: Compensatory gait reflective of quadriceps muscle injury of some kind; characterized by forward flexion of the trunk, forceful plantar flexion of the ankle, and knee hyperextension.
- **Plantar flexion gait**: Compensatory gait due to plantar flexor deficit; distinguished by absent or decreased push-off, shortened stance phase, and short step length on uninvolved side.

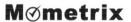

- **Psoatic limp**: Observed in patients with inhibition of the psoas major muscle due to a hip condition like Legg-Calve-Perthes disease; characterized by difficulty in swing phase, limping, and overstated trunk and pelvic movement.

MUSCULOSKELETAL-RELATED LABORATORY TESTS

Bone diseases can often be differentiated by looking in combination at plasma levels of calcium, ionized calcium, inorganic phosphorus, alkaline phosphatase, and phosphorus. Alkaline phosphatase is elevated in most bone diseases, including childhood rickets, adult osteomalacia, Paget's disease, primary hyperparathyroidism, and marked hyperthyroidism. Calcium levels are elevated in primary hyperparathyroidism, multiple myeloma, and Paget's disease (sometimes) but are usually normal in other bone diseases. Samples of synovial fluid can place disease into one of four groups based on appearance:

- **Group 1**: Clear yellow; indicative of noninflammatory conditions or trauma
- **Group 2**: Cloudy; generally due to inflammatory arthritis
- **Group 3**: Brownish with a thick exudate associated with septic arthritis or gout
- **Group 4**: Hemorrhagic; indicates trauma, fractures, bleeding disorders, or tumors

DIAGNOSTIC TESTS FOR MUSCULOSKELETAL EVALUATION

Special diagnostic tests may be used for musculoskeletal/neuromuscular evaluation to confirm a provisional diagnosis, formulate a differential diagnosis, comprehend unusual or difficult signs or symptoms, or differentiate between structures. Any test used must be reliable, sensitive, and specific. Reliability means the test is dependable and can be trusted to measure what is expected. Statistically, reliability can be evaluated in terms of parameters, such as the intraclass correlation coefficient (ICC), which is determined by analysis of variance (ANOVA), with a value > 90 indicating enough agreement for reasonable validity; the kappa, or K statistic, if only nominal data is available; and the standard error of measurement (SEM), which indicates the reliability of response over time and should be small. Sensitivity refers to the ability to detect changes and identify true positives. Specificity is the degree to which the test excludes a particular condition and identifies a true negative. Likelihood ratios combine sensitivity and specificity.

PLAIN FILM RADIOGRAPHY

Two projections using plain film radiography are usually taken: an anteroposterior (AP) and a lateral projection. Others might be taken in special circumstances, such as an oblique view for the lumbar spine. Several projections are needed because of the likelihood of superimposition of structures. Dense structures like metal or bone do not allow penetration of x-rays on the fill and appear relatively white and radiolucent. Less dense structures that allow some penetration like soft tissues (muscles, joint capsules, fat pads, etc.) look grayer, and air spaces that permit complete x-ray penetration are quite black and radiolucent. Fractures, dislocations, and other abnormalities can be visualized. For example, a darker area would be seen where a bone is fractured. Soft tissue injuries are less distinguishable on radiographs and clinical findings are more useful, unless the examiner is extremely adept at interpretation. For musculoskeletal evaluation, the types of things to look for on a radiograph are size, shape, number, alignment, and density of bones; breaks in continuity of the bone; soft-tissue changes, such as swelling or visible fat pads; the width and symmetry of the joint space, etc.

ADDITIONAL DIAGNOSTIC IMAGING INVOLVING RADIATION

One imaging technique involving radiation is arthrography, in which an iodine-containing contrast dye, air, or both are injected into a joint space before taking a radiograph. A variation of this is computed arthrography (CT-arthrography), which merges arthrography with computed

95

tomography (CT), a technique that uses x-ray bombardment from various angles to create a three-dimensional image. Computed tomography can also be used alone and is very useful for assessing cortical bone and identifying spinal stenosis, disc problems, fractures in complex joints, and the like. In myelography, a radiopaque dye is instilled into the epidural space by spinal puncture and a radiograph is taken after diffusion to look at nerve roots and the spinal cord. Venograms and arteriograms use injection of radiopaque dyes into veins and arteries, respectively, to identify conditions, such as blockage after trauma. Discography uses injection of radiopaque dye into the nucleus pulposus of an intervertebral disc. Bone scan, or osteoscintigraphy, use intravenous injection of radioactive tracers (usually technetium-99m labeled); this technique is good at identifying the metabolic status of the skeleton, making it especially useful for detecting skeletal metastases, bone disease, and stress fractures with minimal bone loss, etc.

MAGNETIC RESONANCE IMAGING AND DIAGNOSTIC ULTRASOUND

Unlike most other techniques that involve radiation, magnetic resonance imaging (MRI) and diagnostic ultrasound utilize electromagnetic radiation and high-frequency sound waves, respectively, to create images of bone and soft tissues. MRI utilizes the fact that a strong magnetic field attracts hydrogen atoms. Depending on the type of image taken, MRI is very good for visualization of the anatomy or pathology of soft tissues like muscles and ligaments. It is now preferred over myelography for interpretation of disc pathology.

Diagnostic ultrasound is based on the principle that high-frequency sound waves (5 MHz to 10 MHz) bombarding tissues have a characteristic echo, or return time, depending on the depth of the structure. Diagnostic ultrasound is primarily used to evaluate soft-tissue injury.

Musculoskeletal Diseases/Conditions that Impact Effective Treatment

STRAINS, SPRAINS, AND TENDON INJURIES

Strains are tears in the contractile fibers of the muscles and are defined in terms of the degree of tearing (first degree: few fibers, second degree: approximately half, third degree: all ruptured). They are due to overstretching, overloading, or sometimes crushing. Sprains are tears in ligaments, which are considered inert tissues as they do contract and are not neurologic. The degree of tearing again defines them, similar to strains; they are also due to overload or overstretch. Both strains and sprains are felt acutely; cause pain on stretching, unless third degree; cause moderate to major weakness and swelling, if second or third degree; and decrease range of motion, unless severe, in which case the response depends on swelling. Some differences observed include:

- Muscle spasms are only minor with sprains, but can be much more severe with strains
- Joint play is only excessive in third-degree sprains
- Isometric contractions only produce pain if there is a strain
- Functional losses present differently, for instance, second- and, particularly, third-degree strains or sprains produce reflex inhibition and instability, respectively.

Peritenonitis and tendinosis refer to inflammation and damage to contractile tendons, respectively, as a result of overuse, overstretch, or overload. They tend to be more chronic and may cause crepitus, or popping sounds.

HIP DISLOCATION

Hip dislocations, or displacements, usually develop in a posterior direction, manifesting as a shortened limb, internal rotation, and adduction in slight flexion. They can occur alone or in

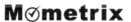

conjunction with a femoral or acetabular fracture. If there is no fracture, hip dislocations are managed with closed reduction and muscle relaxation. If these interventions fail, open reduction or traction is used. If there is associated fracture, surgery is necessary. For patients with hip displacements without fracture, appropriate physical therapy interventions are partial or as tolerated weight-bearing mobility and, depending on the physician's instructions, positioning, and certain exercises.

FRACTURES

DESCRIBING FRACTURES

Fractures are generally described in terms of whether skin integrity is maintained; the site, configuration, and extent of the fracture; and the relative position of the fragments:

- **Bony** fractures are referred to as closed, if the skin is not broken, and open, if there are open tears or bony protrusions.
- The **site** of the fracture refers to its position on the bone, which for long bones would be at the proximal third, distal third, or shaft. Other possible site descriptions include intraarticular and extraarticular, meaning involving or not involving, respectively, the articular surface; and epiphyseal, indicating growth plate involvement.
- The **configuration** is basically orientation of the fracture. Linear fractures are described as transverse (at right angles to the long axis), oblique (diagonal to the long axis), or spiral (also diagonal but more involved with a circular pattern). Configurations where there are two or more fractures are known as comminuted (usually has wedge-shaped fragments) or segmental (at different levels).
- The **extent** is either incomplete or complete, depending on whether one portion or all bone cortices, respectively, are disrupted.
- **Nondisplaced versus displaced** fractures refer respectively to normal or abnormal anatomical alignment of the fracture fragments.

STAGES OF BONE HEALING AFTER FRACTURES

After a fracture, the bone heals in four stages:

1. **Hematoma formation**: Occurs during the first three days after fracture.
2. **Fibrocartilage**: Typically forms within two weeks of the break.
3. **Pro-callus**: Develops during approximately the same time period, about three to 10 days following the break.
4. **Remodeling of the bone or permanent callus formation healing**: Occurs three to 10 weeks after fracture.

Here, the term callus refers to a mass of fibrous tissue, calcium, cartilage, and bone. The healing process is encouraged by factors that include early mobilization and weight bearing, preservation of fracture reduction, and patient compliance. It can be deterred by factors, such as comorbidities like diabetes or anemia, osteoporosis, and disruption of the vascular supply to the affected bone. The extent of soft-tissue damage and the type of fracture affect the healing process; for example, comminuted or multiple fragment fractures take longer to heal.

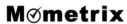

GENERAL FRACTURE MANAGEMENT

Depending on factors such as fracture type and homodynamic stability, fractures are treated as elective, urgent, or emergent.

- **Elective management** usually applies to any type of nonoperative or operative procedure done within days or weeks in a patient whose fracture is stable and neurovascular system normal.
- **Urgent management**, done within one to three days, is a procedure done on a closed but unstable bone in a patient with an intact neurovascular system.
- **Emergent treatments** are those done on open fractures, fractures or dislocations where the neurovascular system is damaged or where there is compartment syndrome, or spinal injuries with neurological defects.

The goal of each is fracture reduction, which is aligning and bringing fragments closer. Methods to achieve fracture reduction are either closed, such as manual manipulation or traction, or open, generally open-reduction internal fixation (ORIF) in which plates, screws, etc., are inserted for immobilization. Otherwise, noninvasive immobilization modalities include casts and splints.

COMPLICATIONS OF FRACTURES

There are many possible complications that can occur shortly after a fracture. Immediate complications within days can include loss of the fixation or reduction, but most are related to other systems and can be critical, including deep vein thrombosis, pulmonary emboli, nerve damage (including paralysis), damage to arteries, compartment syndrome, infection at the incision site, orthostatic hypotension, and shock. Later complications are usually related to the fracture directly, such as its failure to unite within the expected time frame; nonunion; malunion, in which the fracture heals with a deformity; and pseudarthrosis, or formation of a false joint, at the site. Bone-related diseases (such as posttraumatic arthritis, osteomyelitis, or inflammation) or myositis ossificans (where there is bone in the muscle) may develop. These complications are considered delayed or late, depending on whether they appear within weeks to months or later, respectively.

PELVIC RING FRACTURES

ANTEROPOSTERIOR COMPRESSION TYPES

Pelvic ring fractures involve the area of the pelvis fashioned by the paired coxal bone, sacrum, sacroiliac joints, and symphysis pubic. There are three possible anteroposterior compression (APC) types of fractures, all of which involve disruption of the pubic symphysis, as well as lateral compression (LC) and vertical shear fractures:

- **APC, type I**: Shows no other involvement; treated with symptomatic pain management
- **APC, type II**: Involves more than 2.5 cm tearing of the anterior sacroiliac, sacrospinous, and sacrotuberous ligaments; requires exterior fixation or open-reduction internal fixation (ORIF)
- **APC, type III**: Completely interrupts the pubic symphysis, as well as the posterior ligament complexes, and exhibit hemipelvic displacement; may be managed with external fixation, ORIF, or posterior percutaneous pinning

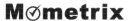

LATERAL COMPRESSION TYPES

Lateral compression (LC) fractures can be of three types:

- **LC, type I** refers to posterior compression of the sacroiliac joint and oblique public ramus fracture, which can be managed with symptomatic pain relief.
- In **LC, type II**, the posterior sacroiliac ligament is also ruptured and the hemipelvis is rotated, requiring external fixation or anterior and posterior open-reduction internal fixation (ORIF).
- **LC, type III** fractures also include an APC or anteroposterior compression injury to the contralateral pelvis, which is managed with anterior and posterior ORIF.

There are also vertical shear fractures, in which a hemipelvis is displaced due to extensive ligament or bone disruption and treated with traction and fixation (percutaneous, external, or anterior and posterior ORIF).

PHYSICAL THERAPY INTERVENTIONS

Appropriate physical therapy interventions depend on the type of pelvic ring fracture. Suitable physical therapy interventions for anteroposterior compression (APC), type I and lateral compression (LC), type I fractures are partial weight bearing (PWB) or weight bearing as tolerated (WBAT) for functional mobility and active/active-assistive range of motion (A/AAROM) of the hip and distal joint. For APC, type II pelvic ring fractures, appropriate interventions are non-weight bearing (NWB), touch-down weight bearing (TDWB), or PWB mobility; hip and distal joint A/AAROM; and lower-extremity exercise. For APC, type III fractures, physical therapy is limited to NWB or TDWB on the least-affected side (basically bed transfers) and A/AAROM on distal lower extremities. These restrictions are also appropriate for LC, types II and III and vertical shear fractures. Patients with vertical shear fractures of the pelvic ring should also do positioning, breathing exercises, and uninvolved extremity exercise if they are on bed rest.

ACETABULAR FRACTURES

The acetabulum is the concave surface on either side of the pelvis where the head of the femur meets the pelvis, forming the hip joint. Acetabular, or hip joint, fractures arise as secondary shocks transmitted from high-impact blunt forces elsewhere, such as a foot with extended knee or the posterior pelvis. Patients with these fractures are prone to other complications, such as hematomas, emboli, and DVT. Fractures are defined as either stable or unstable. A stable acetabular fracture is one where the weight-bearing surface is intact and there is less than 2.5 mm displacement of the dome; these are managed with traction and bed rest and/or closed reduction. An unstable fracture is one in which the weight-bearing dome is fractured, which requires percutaneous pinning, open-reduction internal fixation (ORIF), or total hip arthroplasty. Acetabular fractures are also classified in terms of portion severed, i.e., the anterior or posterior column and transverse or complex (T-shaped), involving both columns. Appropriate physical therapy for stable fractures is touch-down or partial weight bearing, gentle range of motion (ROM), positioning, breathing exercises, and uninvolved breathing exercises if on bed rest. For unstable fractures, partial or as tolerated weight bearing and gentle hip ROM are indicated.

FEMORAL HEAD AND NECK FRACTURES

INTRACAPSULAR

The femur is the main bone in the human thigh; its head and neck are its highest parts in association with the hip. Thus, these fractures are termed hip fractures. They usually occur in the neck portion. They are subdivided into intracapsular and extracapsular fractures, referring to

99

location within or outside the hip capsule, respectively. Intracapsular femoral neck (i.e., hip) fractures have been classified by Garden as follows:

- **Garden I fractures** are impacted but incomplete and can be managed with closed reduction with percutaneous pinning or, rarely, a spica cast.
- **Garden II fractures** are complete fractures without displacement, which is dealt with by closed reduction or open-reduction internal fixation (ORIF).
- **Garden III fractures** are complete with partial displacement but the capsule is partially intact; ORIF is used.
- **Garden IV fractures** are complete with full displacement and capsule disruption; management options include ORIF and univocal or bipolar arthroplasty.

Suggested physical therapy for type I is partial (PWB) or non-weight bearing mobility, active/active-assisted ROM, and lower extremity; similar interventions are used for types II, III, and IV, except for mobility, which should be PWB or as tolerated (for type IV).

EXTRACAPSULAR

Femoral head and neck (i.e., hip) fractures that are outside of the hip capsule are termed extracapsular. Within this taxonomy, there are two types of intertrochanteric (between the greater and lesser trochanters) and four types of subtrochanteric (top portion of femoral shaft) fractures. Intertrochanteric fractures are classified as Evans type I or II, depending on whether the fracture line extends upward or downward from the lesser trochanter. Evans type I is managed with closed-reduction internal fixation or open-reduction internal fixation (ORIF), while options for Evans type II include ORIF, with or without osteotomy and bone grafting, as well as bipolar arthroplasty.

Subtrochanteric fractures are classified as Russell-Taylor types IA, IB, IIA, or IIB. Type A fractures are single, and type B fractures have a second fracture line. In types IA and IB, the only or major line is from below the lesser to the distal greater trichinae, whereas for types IIA and IIB, it extends into the greater trichinae. ORIF is a management option for all. Intramedullary rods are used for types IA, IB, and IIA; dynamic hip screws for types IIA and IIB; and bone grafting for type IIB.

PHYSICAL THERAPY INTERVENTIONS

The appropriate physical therapy interventions for intertrochanteric Evans type I and subtrochanteric Russell-Taylor types IA, IB, or IIA are all similar. They include partial weight bearing for functional mobility, gentle hip range-of-motion (ROM) exercises, and distal lower-extremity strengthening exercises. Comparable ROM and distal lower-extremity exercises can be used for the other types of extracapsular fractures, but weight bearing needs to be more restricted. Touch-down weight bearing (TDWB) is suggested for intertrochanteric Evans type II fractures, and non-weight bearing or TDWB exercises for functional mobility are the only ones that should be used for patients with subtrochanteric Russell-Taylor type IIB fractures.

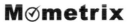
FEMORAL SHAFT FRACTURES

Femoral shaft fractures are generally the result of forceful trauma and can be accompanied by critical complications, such as hypovolemia or shock, hip dislocations, patellar fractures, or abdominal or pelvic injuries. There are three types of femoral fractures:

- **Closed, simple, or nondisplaced**: Managed with open-reduction internal fixation (ORIF) or insertion of an intramedullary rod.
- **Closed, comminuted, impacted, or both**: Can be treated similarly or with traction and bed rest.
- **Open, comminuted, and displaced**: May require irrigation, debridement and wound closure, brief skeletal traction on bed rest, external fixation, and/or an intramedullary rod.

For simple or nondisplaced closed fractures, the suggested physical therapy approach is non-, touch-down, or as tolerated weight bearing for functional mobility, and gentle range-of-motion (ROM) exercises. For the other two types, physical therapy should be limited to non- or touch-down weight bearing, and other interventions should include lower-extremity ROM exercises as directed by the physician, and positioning, breathing exercises, and unaffected-extremity exercises if on bed rest. Single crutches are often used for transfer.

DISTAL FEMORAL FRACTURES

Distal femoral fractures are caused by forceful trauma to the femur or some force that pushes the tibia into the intercondylar fossa. They are often accompanied by local soft-tissue injury. There are five possible types. Two are supracondylar, meaning only the femoral shaft is involved: extraarticular, simple, nondisplaced, for which a long leg cast is indicated; and supracondylar: extraarticular, displaced, or comminuted. Management options for the latter include traction on bed rest, open-reduction internal fixation (ORIF), closed reduction with percutaneous plate fixation, some type of knee immobilizer, an intramedullary nail, and/or passive motion. Fractures that involve one or both condyles are classified as unicondylar or intercondylar, which by definition means they are intraarticular. Unicondylar fractures are divided into non-displaced types, which are managed with a long cast, and displaced types, which require traction on bed rest, ORIF, a long splint or cast, and/or closed-reduction and percutaneous fixation. Intercondylar fractions are treated with long-term traction, ORIF, or a cast brace.

PHYSICAL THERAPY INTERVENTIONS

For supracondylar distal femur fractions that are simple or nondisplaced, the appropriate physical therapy interventions are non-weight bearing mobility and distal and proximal active/active-assisted range-of-motion (A/AAROM) exercises. If the supracondylar fracture is displaced or comminuted, the management is different the patient is often on bed rest. This means positioning, breathing exercises, and unaffected-extremity exercises are indicated, as well as distal and proximal A/AAROM; the type of functional mobility should be partial weight bearing. For nondisplaced unicondylar fractures, physical therapy should include non- or touch-down weight bearing and distal and proximal A/AAROM. Patients with unicondylar fractures with displacement should do touch-down weight bearing, gentle ROM exercise, and continuous passive motion as medically directed. Appropriate physical therapy for patients with intercondylar fractures is touch-down or light partial weight bearing, anything that will maintain functional ROM in the hip and ankle and, eventually, gentle ROM and exercises for the quadriceps.

PATELLAR FRACTURES

The patella, or knee cap bone, articulates with the femur. Patellar fractures are generally caused by direct blows or abrupt quadriceps contractions. There are three common types: nondisplaced,

displaced, and comminuted. Nondisplaced patellar fractures are treated with closed reduction or with a long leg cast or other immobilizer with the knee in full extension. Displaced patellar fractures, either vertical or transverse, are managed with open-reduction internal fixation (ORIF) and continuous passive motion. Appropriate physical therapy interventions for both are partial or as tolerated weight bearing, making sure the fracture is not stressed and, for the displaced type, eventual active-assisted range of motion exercises as directed. Comminuted patellar fractures are managed with ORIF, a partial or total patellectomy with quadriceps tendon repair, or immobilization using a long leg cast or brace or a posterior splint with the knee in full extension or minimal flexion. Functional mobility should be limited to non-, partial, or as tolerated weight bearing, and strong quadriceps contractions should be avoided.

TIBIAL PLATEAU FRACTURES

The tibia or shinbone is the larger of two bones in the lower leg. Blows to the tibial plateau at the apex can be critical since they are often accompanied by open wounds, soft tissue damage, dislocation, nerve compression, deep vein thrombosis, and/or infection. There are three common types. The first is nondisplaced, which is treated with closed reduction, immobilization using a cast or brace, and, if necessary, ligament repair; suggested physical therapy includes touch-down or partial weight bearing and active-assisted range-of-motion (ROM) and/or continuous passive motion. Displaced fractures fall into one of two categories. If the fracture involves a single condyle or split compression, management options are open-reduction internal fixation (ORIF), external fixation, and/or a cast or brace; physical therapy is the same as for nondisplaced fractures described above. For displaced fractures that are impacted or significantly comminuted involving both condyles, the management options are skeletal traction with bed rest, ORIF with or without bone grafting, an immobilization brace, and, if necessary. ligament or meniscus repair. Only non-, touch-down, or partial weight bearing should be done along with positioning, breathing and uninvolved-extremity exercises (if on bed rest), and, eventually, knee A/AAROM.

TIBIAL SHAFT AND FIBULA FRACTURES

The tibia and fibula are the large and small calf bones, respectively. Fractures occur through direct impact, stress at the knee, or twisting of the ankle. They may be accompanied by ankle fractures, damage to the tibial artery or peroneal nerve, or rupture of the interosseous membrane. There are three classifications of closed tibial shaft fractures and one open type. Closed tibial shaft fractures are described as minimally displaced, which require closed reduction or a long leg cast; moderately displaced, managed with open-reduction internal fixation (ORIF) or a short leg cast; or severely displaced, comminuted, or both, requiring external fixation, ORIF, and/or provisional calcaneal (heel bone) traction. Open tibial shaft fractures are managed with ORIF or external fixation.

Appropriate physical therapy interventions for minimally displaced closed fractures are touch-down, partial, or as tolerated weight bearing, quadriceps strengthening, and edema control. With moderate displacement, only non- or touch-down weight bearing should be done, along with knee range-of-motion (ROM) exercises, quadriceps strengthening, and edema management. Severely displaced or comminuted closed or open fractures should be addressed with ankle and possibly knee ROM exercises, quadriceps strengthening, and edema control.

DISTAL TIBIAL FRACTURES

Distal tibial fractures generally occur from falls or other vertical loading forces, often in association with ankle fractures. There are three types of closed tibial fractures, based on degree of displacement, and one open type. The closed distal tibial fractures are described as: minimally displaced, which are managed with closed reduction or a short leg cast; moderately displaced, treated with open-reduction internal fixation (ORIF) or a short leg cast; or severely displaced, requiring temporary traction of the calcaneus (heel bone), external fixation, and/or ORIF. Open distal tibial fractures require external fixation.

The appropriate physical therapy interventions for patients with minimally or moderately displaced distal tibial fractures are non-weight bearing functional mobility, knee range of motion (ROM) exercises, strengthening of the proximal joint, and edema control. For those with severely displaced closed fractures, lower-extremity isometrics and neutral ankle positioning should be done instead of knee ROM. For open fractures, ankle ROM exercises and neutral ankle positioning are substituted.

ANKLE FRACTURES

Ankle fractures are usually due to torque from abnormal loading of the talocrural joint, which connects the tibia and fibula to the talus bone of the foot. There are three possible types:

- **Closed, nondisplaced fractures** are addressed with closed reduction and a short leg or walking cast; appropriate physical therapy is non- or partial weight bearing functional mobility, exercises to strengthen the proximal lower extremity, and edema management.
- **Closed fractures** that are displaced and/or multifractured are managed via closed reduction, open-reduction internal fixation (ORIF), and a cast or other type of mobilization depending on the amount of edema.
- **Open ankle fractures** are treated with irrigation and debridement with wound closure, traction, external fixation, and/or ORIF.

In the latter two cases, the suggested physical therapy regimen is non-weight bearing mobility; proximal lower-extremity strengthening; foot and ankle exercises, as prescribed by the physician; and edema control.

CALCANEAL FRACTURES

Calcaneal fractures are those occurring in the calcaneus, or heel bone. They usually occur from high falls or sometimes avulsion, are often bilateral, and may be associated with leg or spinal fractures. There are four types of calcaneal injuries:

- **Extraarticular**, minimally displaced, which is managed with closed reduction and a short leg cast (SLC)
- **Avulsion**, with management options of closed reduction, a SLC, and open-reduction internal fixation (ORIF)
- **Intraarticular**, involving the subtalar joint (foot joint between calcaneus and talus), which is managed with skeletal traction, a SLC, ORIF, closed reduction with percutaneous pinning, and/or arthrodesis, if the fracture is extensive
- **Open**, which requires irrigation and debridement with wound closure, skeletal traction, and/or external fixation

The suggested physical therapy regimen for patients with any of these calcaneal fractures is non-weight bearing functional mobility; strengthening and range of motion exercises for the proximal lower extremity; ankle and forefoot exercises, as prescribed by the physician; and edema management.

FOREFOOT FRACTURES

The forefoot, or metatarsal bones, includes the five bones connected to the toes. Forefoot fractures are a result of objects falling on the foot, twisting, stress, or avulsion. There are three possible types of forefoot fractures:

- **Minimally displaced**, which is treated with closed reduction, percutaneous pinning, and/or a short leg or walking cast.
- **Moderate to severely displaced** with fragmentation or angulation, managed with open-reduction internal fixation (ORIF), a short leg cast, and/or percutaneous pinning.
- **Open**, which requires irrigation and debridement with wound closure, skeletal traction, external fixation, and/or ORIF.

The suggested physical therapy interventions are the same for any of these types, namely proximal lower-extremity strengthening and range of motion, edema management, and, depending on the location and severity of the fracture, non-, partial, or as tolerated weight bearing mobility.

SPINAL FRACTURES

Common causes of spinal fractures are vehicle accidents, falls, sports injuries, and violence. Spinal fractures are defined in terms of their location, as involving the anterior column and/or posterior column.

- The **anterior column** of the spine includes the vertebral bodies, intervertebral discs, and the anterior and posterior longitudinal ligaments.
- The **posterior column** includes the transverse and spinous processes, pedicles and laminae of the vertebral arch, and various ligaments.

Spinal fractures are also described in terms of whether they are stable or unstable. A stable fracture involves only one column (anterior or posterior) or is one lacking neurologic insufficiency. Spinal fractures are differentiated in terms of area of the spine affected, as cervical or thoracolumbar. Potential complications of spinal fractures include swelling at the site, hematomas, herniation or dislocation of the intervertebral disc, and spinal cord injury. Therefore, the patient must be closely monitored for other fractures, head and internal injuries, neurovascular parameters, and, in the case of cervical fractures, airway and breathing.

CERVICAL SPINE FRACTURES

Cervical spine fractures are bone breaks in the neck region. There are basically four types of cervical spine fractures, some of which are further differentiated. Two stable types are vertebral body fractures, which are wedge fractures involving bony impaction and concavity of the vertebral body; and isolated spinous process, or laminal fractures. Both types are managed with a cervical collar. Other categories include bilateral pedicle (Hangman's) fractures of axis C1 and odontoid process fractures. Hangman's fractures can be type I (no angulation, minimal displacement), II (displacement), IIA (minimal displacement, significant angulation), or III (full facet dislocation). Management includes cervical collar immobilization for type I, cervical traction/reduction and later a halo vest for types II or IIA, and posterior open reduction with halo vest or C1-3 fusion for type III. Odontoid process fractures are divided into: type I, oblique avulsion fractures at the tip of the odontoid, simply requiring a cervical collar for immobilization; type II, fractures in the neck of the odontoid, treated with closed reduction, ORIF with halo vest, or C1-2 fusion with or without bone grafting and cervical collar; and type III, fractures that extend to C2 vertebral body, managed with closed reduction or ORIF with halo vest.

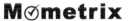

PHYSICAL THERAPY INTERVENTIONS

Patients with stable vertebral body fractures, or isolated spinous process (laminal) fractures, require only functional mobility, posture training, and body mechanics. Those with Hangman's (bilateral pedicle) fractures or odontoid process cervical spine fractures, which are more serious, should be approached differently. For these patients, the appropriate physical therapy interventions include posture and body mechanics training; therapeutic and active assisted/passive range-of-motion exercises, tailored to the neurologic injury; balance and scapular exercises, if they wear a halo vest; and functional mobility with logroll precautions. Logroll precautions mean turning the patient in bed so that the head and torso are a unit.

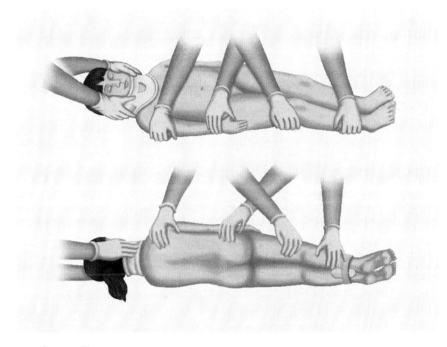

THORACOLUMBAR SPINE FRACTURES

Thoracolumbar spine fractures, those occurring below the cervical region, are divided into four types. The first type is a stable, isolated fracture of a spinous process, transverse process, lamina, or facet, which is managed with a cervicothoracic or thoracolumbar orthosis. There are two types of vertebral body fractures: stable vertebral body compression (impacted anterior wedge) fractures, which are managed with temporary bed rest, vertebroplasty, orthoses, hyperextension braces, or, if severe, fusion; and unstable vertebral body burst (axial compression) fractures, which are addressed with short-term bed rest, orthoses, and anterior/posterior decompression and reconstruction, possibly with bone grafting. The last type of thoracolumbar spine fracture is an unstable multidirectional fracture with disc involvement and facet dislocation, which is managed using anterior/posterior decompression and fusion and an orthosis. Regardless of type, the appropriate physical therapy interventions are functional mobility with logroll precautions, postural and body mechanic training, and therapeutic exercise and active-assisted passive range of motion as indicated by the neurologic injury.

SHOULDER GIRDLE FRACTURES

The areas of possible fracture on the shoulder girdle are primarily the glenohumeral (shoulder) joint, the coracoid process of the scapula, the clavicle (collar bone), and the scapula (bone connecting the arm bone and clavicle). Stable, nondisplaced fractures of the glenohumeral or coracoid regions are treated conservatively with sling immobilization. If there is displacement, they

105

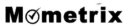

are managed with open-reduction internal fixation (ORIF). Acute management for glenohumeral dislocation is closed reduction to avert neurovascular damage. Clavicle fractures are managed conservatively with a sling unless there are complications, such as neurovascular damage, ligament tears, or a floating shoulder, in which case ORIF is indicated. Scapular fractures are uncommon due to muscular protection, and pain management is usually sufficient.

PROXIMAL HUMERAL FRACTURES

The humerus is the long bone of the upper arm. Proximal humeral fractures are due to some type of trauma and primarily occur in the greater tuberosity. Most proximal humeral fractures are nondisplaced or minimally displaced, which would be treated conservatively. Proximal fractures that are displaced are described in terms of the number of parts. One-part displaced proximal humeral fractures are managed with closed reduction or sling immobilization, and two-part ones are managed with closed reduction and percutaneous pinning, open-reduction internal fixation (ORIF), an intramedullary rod, or a sling. If the displaced fracture is three parts, the management options are hemiarthroplasty and ORIF; four-part fractures are treated with transcutaneous reduction with fluoroscopy, percutaneous pinning, or ORIF. Another possibility is comminution of the humeral head, which is managed with hemiarthroplasty and sling immobilization. Suggested physical therapy for any of these types of fractures is non-weight bearing functional mobility, pendulum exercises and passive range of motion (ROM) as prescribed, edema control, and ROM exercises for the elbow, wrist, and hand.

HUMERAL SHAFT FRACTURES

Humeral shaft fractures are generally one of three types:

- **Closed with minimal displacement**: Managed with closed reduction, a sling, hanging arm cast, or brace.
- **Closed, displaced with angulation**: Requires open-reduction internal fixation (ORIF), an intramedullary rod, or a long arm splint.
- **Open**: Necessitates irrigation and debridement with wound closure, external fixation, and/or ORIF.

Regardless of type, the appropriate physical therapy interventions include non-weight bearing functional mobility, isometric scapulothoracic exercises, wrist and hand exercises, edema control, and shoulder and elbow active/active-assisted range of motion drills as prescribed by the physician based on the type of immobilization.

DISTAL HUMERAL AND OLECRANON FRACTURES

Distal humeral and olecranon fractures are in the elbow region. Distal humeral refers to the portion of the humerus near the elbow, the olecranon (elbow bone) is the upper portion of the ulna (larger forearm bone), and the radial head is the uppermost portion of the radius (smaller forearm bone). Most distal humeral fractures are intercondylar T- or Y-shaped or, for the elderly, transcondylar. Stable distal humeral fractures are managed with immobilization and early range-of-motion (ROM) exercises; comminuted intraarticular ones require open-reduction internal fixation (ORIF) or total elbow arthroplasty (TEA). Management options for closed olecranon fractures depend on the whether they are nondisplaced (a long arm cast with the elbow in midflexion), displaced (ORIF), or comminuted (ORIF and immobilization). Severely comminuted olecranon fractures are usually found in conjunction with humeral fracture and elbow dislocation. The appropriate physical therapy regimen for any olecranon fracture is non-weight bearing functional mobility, distal and proximal joint active ROM, edema management, and elbow active-assisted ROM that is not painful, per physician order.

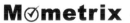

RADIAL HEAD FRACTURES

The radial head is the uppermost portion of the radius, the smaller forearm bone. Radial head fractures lie in the elbow region. Closed radial head or neck fractures, which are generally associated with elbow dislocation and various soft-tissue disruptions, are managed according to degree of displacement. If the radial head is nondisplaced or minimally displaced, the fracture is managed with closed reduction with early immobilization, a sling or temporary splint, and aspiration of the associated hematoma, if necessary. Treatments for displaced closed radial head fractures include partial or complete excision of the radial head, closed reduction and short-term splinting for those with sufficient range of motion (ROM), and open-reduction internal fixation (ORIF) for people with inadequate ROM. Comminuted closed radial head fractures are managed with ORIF with immobilization and radial head excision with or without a radial head prosthesis and bone grafting. The appropriate physical therapy regimen for any radial head fracture is non-weight bearing functional mobility, distal and proximal joint active ROM, edema management, and elbow active-assisted ROM that is not painful, per physician order.

FOREARM FRACTURES

The larger and shorter bones in the forearm are the ulna and radius, respectively. Most of these fractures are displaced, affecting contiguous articulation; and the humerus or wrist is often fractured as well. Fractures affecting the shaft of either the ulna or radius are managed with casting and, if displaced, closed reduction, or open-reduction internal fixation (ORIF) with a functional brace. Distal radius fractures generally fall into one of three types:

- Extraarticular: Treated with closed reduction with percutaneous pinning; ORIF, with or without a functional brace; or a sugar-tong splint or cast.
- Intraarticular: Managed with options that include ORIF; closed reduction with external fixation and, possibly, percutaneous pinning; or arthroscopic internal fixation
- Intraarticular, comminuted: Requires closed reduction with external fixation, ORIF, bone grafting, and/or a splint

Suggested physical therapy for all of these forearm fractures includes non-weight bearing functional mobility, distal and proximal range-of-motion exercises, and edema control. In addition, intraarticular radius fractures (including comminuted ones) indicate use of active and passive movements if the patient has external fixation.

CARPAL, METACARPAL, AND PHALANGEAL FRACTURES

The carpal, metacarpal, and phalangeal (phalanx) bones are located, respectively, just above the wrist crease, in the palm, and in the fingers of the hand. Each term represents a number of bones.

- Carpal fractures are usually due to compression or hyperextension injuries, and there is generally associated ligament damage or dislocation. The management for nondisplaced carpal fractures is a short arm cast with the wrist held neutral with slight ulnar deviation; for displaced fractures, it is closed reduction and casting or open-reduction internal fixation (ORIF) with a splint or cast.
- Metacarpal fractures occur subsequent to direct trauma or weight on the long axis, and there may be associated soft-tissue damage. The fracture location determines treatment: ORIF for the articular surface; closed reduction, percutaneous pinning, and/or immobilization, if the fracture is in the neck or shaft; or percutaneous pinning and immobilization for base metacarpal fractures.

- Phalangeal fractures are most often caused by direct force to the hand, such as crushing, which usually also affects soft tissues. Phalangeal fractures are treated with reduction and splinting, if nondisplaced, or ORIF with splinting, if displaced or intraarticular.

SPINAL DEFORMITIES
LORDOSIS

Lordosis is a common spinal deformity in which there is abnormal forward curvature of the spine in the lumbar and cervical regions. Among its causes are postural or functional deformities, compensation for another deformity like kyphosis, and lax abdominal or other muscles in combination with tight muscles (particularly the hip flexors or lumbar extensors). People with pathological lordosis have postural abnormalities developed as compensation to maintain the proper center of gravity, such as drooping shoulders, medial rotation of the legs, hyperextended knees, slight plantar flexion in the ankle joints, and forward thrusting of the head. Their pelvic angle is increased from the normal 30-40°, putting them in an anterior pelvic tilt; they develop stress on many joints; many of their muscles are elongated and weak, particularly the deep lumbar extensors; and other muscles are tight, such as the hip flexors. Swayback deformity is similar in that there is a 40° pelvic inclination, but there is posterior spinal curvature in the thoracolumbar region and the hip joint is pushed forward. People with swayback generally have weak hip flexors, lower abdominals, and lower thoracic extensors; and tight hip extensors, upper abdominals, and lower lumber extensors.

KYPHOSIS

Kyphosis is exaggerated posterior curvature of the spine in the thoracic region. Causes of kyphosis include vertebral compression fractures, osteoporosis, tumors, congenital defects, and compensation for lordosis, paralysis, and Scheuermann's vertebral osteochondritis. The latter is a common disease in which there is inflammation of bone and cartilage in the ring epiphysis of the vertebral body. There are four varieties of kyphosis:

- **Round back**: A long, rounded, curved back.
- **Flat back**: A mobile lumbar spine, making the spine appear very flat.
- **Humpback** (also called gibbus): A sharp posterior angulation in a small portion of the thoracic spine.
- **Dowager's hump**: The degeneration of thoracic vertebral bodies due to osteoporosis.

People with round, flat, or humpback all have decreased pelvic inclination (approximately 20°). Dowager's hump manifests as loss of height, forward flexion of the head, and protruding abdomen, resulting from the attempt to maintain normal center of gravity. Each of these types is associated with stress on certain joints, poor body alignment, and characteristic elongated, weak and short, strong muscles. Abnormal thoracic and lumbar spine curvatures can result in kypholordotic posture.

SCOLIOSIS

Scoliosis is abnormal curvature of the spine in a lateral direction. Depending on the cause, scoliosis is considered either nonstructural (functional), due to things like postural issues, inflammation, nerve root irritation, or compensation; or structural, due to bone deformities or muscle weakness. The vast majority of structural scoliosis cases are idiopathic, in which there is rotation and distortion of the vertebral bodies. Other causes of structural scoliosis include upper or lower motor neuron lesions, muscular diseases, trauma, and conditions responsible for bone destruction. Nonstructural scoliosis is not progressive, and the individual can flex forward, reducing the

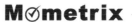

abnormal curvature; whereas structural scoliosis is progressive, the person is relatively inflexible, and side bending is asymmetrical.

CONTRACTURES

A contracture is adaptive shortening or hypomobility of the skin, fascia, muscle, or joint capsule, resulting in decreased mobility or flexibility of the structure. Contractures are usually described in terms of the affected shortened muscle, for example, shortening of the elbow flexor, which would be an elbow flexion contracture. They are also often identified in terms of the pathology, as either myostatic (no specific muscle pathology), pseudomyostatic (due to spasticity or rigidity associated with nervous system disorders), arthrogenic (intraarticular pathology), periarticular (involving associated connective tissues), fibrotic (due to fibrotic changes in connective tissue), and irreversible (usually stemming from fibrotic types).

MUSCULOSKELETAL SURGICAL INTERVENTIONS

HIP ARTHROPLASTY

Arthroplasty, commonly known as joint replacement, is the surgical repair of a joint or its total or partial replacement with metal (titanium, cobalt alloys, etc.) or plastic (generally polyethylene) parts. Hip arthroplasty is typically total hip arthroplasty (THA), in which the femoral head and the acetabulum are both replaced. THA is done in patients with hip disorders, such as degenerative or rheumatoid arthritis, posttraumatic disorders in the area, a fused hip, bone tumors, etc. Usually, the components are uncemented, especially in young or active patients; these have sections of porous coated metal, often treated with hydroxyapatite to encourage bony ingrowth and fixation, or press-fit prostheses that are used to attain fixation. Cemented prostheses are generally only used in patients who cannot regenerate bone effectively, such as those with osteoporosis. If the patient has bone or muscle issues that might cause dislocation, a bipolar cup that snaps over the femoral prosthesis might be used. Surgical approaches for THA combine surgery (posterior, anterior, lateral, or anterolateral) with removal and reattachment of the greater trochanter of the femur.

PHYSICAL THERAPY INTERVENTIONS IMMEDIATELY FOLLOWING HIP ARTHROPLASTY

The main concern of the therapist is to help the patient attain safe functional mobility in areas such as bed mobility, transfers, and walking with assistive devices. Some patients may qualify for early mobilization (getting out of bed 6 hours postoperatively) while others may require 1-2 days of mobilization in the bed to strengthen atrophied muscles prior to ambulation. These decisions should be patient-specific and are generally outlined by the surgeon. Precautions are approach-specific, but generally speaking the patient should be advised not to bend their hip more than 90° or cross their affected leg over the other.

Generally speaking, the patient should lie flat on their back part of the time to stretch the anterior hip muscles. To facilitate transfers, the bed height may need to be raised and elevated and seating surfaces, such hip and commode chairs, may need to be used. The patient will probably need to wear a shoe on the uninvolved side at first to accommodate for a phenomenon known as "apparent leg length discrepancy" resulting from the inserted hardware. Physical therapy should include passive and active-assisted range of motion, which may require an overhead frame with sling. In order to restore control of the quadriceps and peroneal muscles, reduce muscle spasms, and protect the associated femoral and sciatic nerves, a knee immobilizer and/or ankle-foot orthosis may be needed and isometric exercises for these muscles should be instituted after surgery. Eventually, active-assisted exercises for these muscles are indicated as tolerated. Another area of concern is prevention of DVT and edema, which should be addressed with ankle-pumping exercises, compression stockings or devices, and repetitive sets of quadriceps and gluteus exercises.

OUTPATIENT PHYSICAL THERAPY INTERVENTIONS

The initial stages of outpatient rehabilitation following total hip arthroplasty are dependent upon the surgical technique, potential complications, and the findings at the initial evaluation. Patient education regarding any postoperative precautions is paramount. Postoperative hip precautions are dependent upon the surgical approach. The focus of the early phase of rehabilitation is on controlling symptoms, reducing edema, monitoring for signs of infection and deep venous thrombosis (DVT), regaining ROM, and gait training. The patient will work to regain functional mobility in and out of the home with appropriate assistive devices, as needed. Over the course of care the focus of rehabilitation will be on improving ROM, improving lower quarter strength, and returning to all functional daily activities and applicable work tasks. Discharge typically occurs once the patient has maximized their gains with range of motion, strength, and performance of ADLs and applicable work tasks.

JOINT RESURFACING

Joint resurfacing is generally used in patients who have osteonecrosis of the femoral head, instead of total hip arthroplasty (THA). There are two possible joint resurfacing techniques: hemi-resurfacing arthroplasty, in which an adjusted cup is implanted, preserving most of the bone; or total joint resurfacing, in which both the femoral head and acetabulum are resurfaced with a double cup. The physical therapy regimen for patients with joint resurfacing is in many respects similar to that for THA, namely emphasis on mobility, transfers, hip range of motion (ROM), quadriceps strengthening, and gait training. Early mobilization (with assistive devices such as crutches or a walker) is encouraged. These patients can only tolerate partial weight bearing for the first four to six weeks. They should avoid bending beyond 90° at the hip, crossing legs, twisting during exercise, or doing anything else restricted by the physician. Some patients who have joint resurfacing eventually need a THA.

KNEE ARTHROPLASTY

Knee arthroplasty, or replacement, is done to relieve pain or restore joint stability and function. Patients generally have some form of arthritis (rheumatoid, traumatic, or osteoarthritis) or joint disease. There are two types. The first is unicompartmental knee arthroscopy (UKA, also known as unicondylar or partial knee arthroscopy), in which the femoral and tibial articulating surfaces in only one joint compartment (the lateral or medial) are replaced and much of the joint is preserved. The other is tricompartmental or total knee arthroplasty (TKA), in which prosthetics (metal, plastic, etc.) are used to replace the medial and lateral compartments and resurface the patellofemoral articulation (usually). TKA fixation techniques are comparable to those used in hip replacements: cemented or uncemented porous ingrowth or press-fit. Possible complications include thrombosis or embolism, joint instability, damage to the peroneal nerve, patellar tendon rupture, and others.

PHYSICAL THERAPY INTERVENTIONS POST-KNEE ARTHROPLASTY

Immediately post-operatively, physical therapy should be initiated in patients who have undergone knee arthroplasty. The therapy regimen should emphasize bed mobility quickly progressing to out of bed mobility, positioning, edema control, transfer techniques, gait training with appropriate assistive devices, strengthening of the quadriceps with active-assisted exercises, passive or active-assisted range of motion (ROM) up to a flexion of 90° (during the first 2 weeks), and antiembolic exercises. Antiembolic exercises to promote venous circulation and isometric strengthening should consist of quadriceps and gluteus exercises and ankle pumps. The involved limb should be elevated at the foot with pillows, towel rolls, or, if possible, without them to prevent contractures. A pillow or towel roll should also be put under the knee during isometric exercises. A towel roll or blanket placed along the lateral aspect of the femur is useful for maintaining a neutral position. Active-

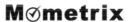

assisted ROM exercises are best done using hold-and-relax techniques to minimize muscle guarding. Ice is generally applied after exercises to reduce edema.

OUTPATIENT PHYSICAL THERAPY INTERVENTIONS

The initial stages of outpatient rehabilitation following total knee arthroplasty are dictated by the surgical technique, postoperative complications, and the findings at the initial evaluation. Patient education regarding signs and symptoms of infection and DVT is key. The priorities of the early phase of rehabilitation are pain management, edema reduction, monitoring for signs of infection and DVT, improving ROM, and gait training in various contexts. The patient will work to regain functional mobility in and out of the home with appropriate assistive devices, as needed. Over the course of care, the focus of rehabilitation will be on attaining at least 115° of flexion and 0° of extension ROM, improving lower quarter strength, and returning to all functional daily activities and applicable work tasks. Discharge typically occurs once the patient has either met all functional goals set in their plan of care or maximized their objective gains with relevant impairments, performance of ADLs, and tolerance of applicable work tasks.

MINIMALLY INVASIVE HIP AND KNEE ARTHROPLASTIES

Minimally invasive surgery (MIS) for a hip or knee arthroplasty is commonplace today for joint replacements or revisions that are less complex. MIS can be done open or arthroscopically using an endoscope. The biggest advantages of MIS hip arthroplasty are that it can be done from the anterior or posterior side and healing is much faster than normal THA. MIS knee arthroscopy involves a much smaller incision than other techniques and minimizes untoward effects like muscle compromise and joint dislocation. Physical therapy for MIS arthroplasties should emphasize maximal functional mobility and is fairly similar to that for those treated by less conservative techniques. Weight bearing as tolerated is usually possible directly after surgery. The key to rapid recovery after MIS or any total joint arthroplasty is early introduction of ambulation (as soon as three hours post-operatively) and other exercises, often in conjunction with short-acting spinal analgesics.

SHOULDER ARTHROPLASTY

Shoulder arthroplasty is performed in patients with various types of arthritis (rheumatoid, traumatic, or osteoarthritis), fractures, or avascular necrosis (AVN) to alleviate pain and restore functionality. There are several types of shoulder arthroplasty. The least invasive is proximal humeral hemiarthroplasty, which is prosthetic replacement of the humeral head, if that is the only portion affected. With more damage, some type of total shoulder arthroplasty (TSA) is done, in which the glenoid articulating surface and humeral head are both prosthetically replaced. Most TSA prostheses are unconstrained, and if there is some damage to the rotator cuff or deltoid muscles, they are repaired during the surgery. Most TSA fixations are cemented or press-fit. Cemented glenoid fixations often lead to loosening, thus requiring revisions. Alternatives include shoulder surface replacement arthroplasty (hemiarthroplasty) and reverse total arthroplasty (Delta III), which shifts the center of rotation and relies primarily on the deltoid muscles for stability, making it good for situations where there is extensive rotator cup damage.

PHYSICAL THERAPY INTERVENTIONS POST-SHOULDER ARTHROPLASTY

The physical therapy interventions for patients who have undergone shoulder arthroplasty are fairly similar regardless of procedure (total shoulder arthroscopy, humeral hemiarthroplasty, shoulder surface replacement arthroplasty, or reverse total arthroplasty). The patient should be instructed not to put weight on the surgically altered extremity, including rolling onto it or lifting anything heavier than a coffee cup. While lying down, the arm should be kept neutral (using a pillow or towel) and not permitted to extend past midline. If they wear an abduction brace for stability, they should be instructed as to how to take it on and off for exercise or dressing. Sling use should only be temporary. The types of physical therapy exercises to include are pendulum exercises in all four planes of motion; gentle passive or active-assisted range of motion (ROM); forward elevation in the scapular plane as tolerated; limited external rotation; active abduction and flexion per physician order; and hand, wrist, and elbow ROM to control edema. The latter ROM exercises should be done with elevation and ice packs. Patients who have had reverse total arthroscopy should be immobilized in slight abduction and neutral rotation.

OUTPATIENT PHYSICAL THERAPY INTERVENTIONS

The initial stages of outpatient rehabilitation following shoulder arthroplasty are dependent upon the surgical technique, potential complications, and the findings at the initial examination. Patient education regarding postoperative precautions as well as the surgeon's instructions regarding the arm sling are paramount. The focus of the early phase of rehabilitation is on controlling symptoms, monitoring for signs of infection, reducing edema, gently restoring PROM and then AAROM of the shoulder, restoring AROM of the distal upper extremity, and performing modified ADLs. The intermediate phase of rehabilitation focuses on continuing to restore PROM, beginning to progress AROM of the shoulder, and addressing scapular stability. The final phases of rehabilitation focus on continuing to improve range of motion while regaining shoulder strength and endurance to allow for the completion of functional ADLs and/or work tasks. Discharge typically occurs once the patient has maximized their outcome related to range of motion, strength, ADL tolerance, and work task tolerance, if applicable.

TOTAL ELBOW ARTHROPLASTY

Total elbow arthroplasty (TEA) is used to relieve pain and promote joint range of motion (ROM) and stability, primarily in rheumatoid arthritis patients. Semiconstrained prostheses of metal and polyethylene with a locking pin or snap-fit device are predominantly used. Other TEA procedures include unconstrained and resurfacing arthroplasties. Fixation designs may be cemented, uncemented, or a combination of the two. Potential complications include loosening, joint instability, weakness of the triceps, ulnar nerve palsy, slow wound healing, and infections (addressed elsewhere). Appropriate physical therapy includes functional mobility and activities of daily life training; edema management; ROM exercises, as prescribed; and if accessible, continuous passive motion to the elbow.

TOTAL ANKLE ARTHROPLASTY

Total ankle arthroplasty is infrequently used in patients with unbearable arthritic pain, primarily in relatively healthy older individuals with low physical demands. The most successful prosthetic designs have been two of the semiconstrained type, both of which are made of metal alloy and polyethylene components and use bony ingrowth for fixation. Potential complications of total ankle arthroplasty include loosening, wound infections, and subtler and midtarsal degenerative joint disease. To avert wound complications after surgery, the patient wears a short leg splint before suture removal and does not do any weight bearing until bony ingrowth is complete, which is about three weeks. Appropriate physical therapy is non-weight bearing functional mobility; edema management; and ankle range of motion and hip and knee strengthening, as ordered.

COMPLICATIONS OF JOINT ARTHROPLASTIES

Infection of the area of a total joint arthroplasty is indicated by fever, wound drainage, unrelenting pain, and abnormally high laboratory values for infection markers, such as white blood cell counts, erythrocyte sedimentation rate, and C-reactive protein. Typically, the joint is aspirated, the fluid is analyzed to isolate the responsible organism, and effective antibiotics prescribed. Irrigation and debridement of the joint area, primary exchange arthroplasty, a two-stage reimplantation or

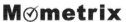

resection, and, possibly, amputation may also be required. A total joint arthroplasty resection involves removal of all previous work, six weeks of IV antibiotics, and then reimplantation of joint components. Two-step resections of the hip or knee include an initial resection of the prosthetic, plus insertion of a cement spacer saturated with antibiotic, and, later, reimplantation.

RESECTION ARTHROPLASTIES POST-JOINT ARTHROPLASTY INFECTION

Resection arthroplasty and two-stage reimplantation are procedures commonly performed after a joint arthroplasty region has become infected. During the healing period, physical therapy should primarily address functional mobility, safety, use of assistive devices, retention of muscle strength and endurance, positioning to reduce muscle spasms, and edema control with ice and elevation. Patients who originally had a total hip or knee arthroplasty are usually less restricted during the period of prosthesis removal and can do most isometric, active, and active-assisted exercises. For knee resection patients before reimplantation, range-of-motion exercises should be kept to a minimum to preserve integrity of bone surfaces. As these patients are non-weight bearing, gait can be assisted by wearing a shoe on the uninvolved side and a slipper sock on the involved side, unless there is leg-length discrepancy in patient with a hip arthroplasty, in which case the foot coverings are reversed.

TOTAL FEMUR REPLACEMENT

Total femur replacement is generally done in patients with advanced malignant sarcoma with extracompartmental involvement. The exact procedure is tailored to the patient, but in general, it entails disarticulation of the hip and knee joints, dissection and ligation of the femoral artery and vein, removal of the entire femur and contiguous musculature, osteotomy of the trochanter bones, insertion of a prosthetic femur secured at the two joints, and wiring of the trochanters into the prosthetic. The procedure permits range of motion at both joints. Suggested physical therapy includes toe touch or non-weight bearing, bed mobility, gait and balance instruction, crutch or walker training, and strength and endurance exercise, including upper extremities, which will need to be used.

HIP DISARTICULATION AND HEMIPELVECTOMY

Hip disarticulation and hemipelvectomy are treatment options for malignant soft-tissue or bone tumors in the hip area. Hip disarticulation entails release of crucial pelvic and hip musculature, dislocation of the hip joint, division of the ligaments, and removal of the extremity. Hemipelvectomy is normally also an amputation of the limb, which is more extensive in that more of the pelvis and, at the end, more of the lower extremity is removed. In young patients with a promising prognosis, a limb-sparing alternative is internal hemipelvectomy, which is usually achieved by additional internal fixation and/or total hip arthroplasty. Patients who have had a leg amputated are potentially plagued by complications, such as infection, phantom pain, orthostatic hypotension, and blood loss. They usually have an attached drain to collect lost blood. Physical therapy should emphasize bed mobility, including learning to sit up; transfer training; gait and balance instruction; crutch or walker training; and functional strength and endurance, including upper extremities, which will need to be used. A good method of transfer is a reclining wheelchair. Patients who have undergone an internal hemipelvectomy can be started on limited weight bearing mobility and joint motion.

TIBIAL AND TROCHANTERIC OSTEOTOMIES

An osteotomy is a surgical procedure in which a bone is divided or sectioned. Tibial osteotomy is a conservative substitute for total knee arthroplasty that maintains the joint by resection of the proximal tibia. Typical post-operative physical therapy includes bed mobility, transfer training, balance and gait instruction, toe-touch weight bearing, active knee range of motion (ROM), and involved extremity strengthening exercises (ankle pumps, quad and gluteus sets). Eventually, the patient should progress to partial weight bearing, then full weight bearing, and additional extremity strengthening exercises, such as active-assisted straight leg raises, hip abduction/adduction, and heel slides.

Trochanteric osteotomy is an adjunct to surgical fixation of a hip fracture or total hip replacement. It involves excision of the greater trochanter, leaving intact musculature, and reattachment of the trochanter to the femur with screws after fixation. Appropriate physical therapy includes toe-touch weight bearing; gait and transfer training, including use of the assistive device; ROM and modest strengthening of the involved hip; bed mobility; antiembolic exercises (ankle pumps, etc. as above); and global strengthening and endurance, particularly with upper extremities, which will be used.

SPINAL SURGERIES

Spinal surgeries are indicated for disabling back pain that is unresponsive to more conservative measures, such as bed rest, anti-inflammatory drugs, lifestyle changes, or physical therapy. Common spinal surgeries include:

- **Discectomy or microdiscectomy**: Removal of the herniated portion or the entire intervertebral disc in patients with herniated nucleus pulpous (HNP).
- **Spinal fusion**: Union of facet joints in the spine with hardware or bone grafting; many types are often done in combination with nerve root decompression surgeries; several indications, including segmental instability, fractures, and arthritis of the facet joints.
- **Laminectomy**: Removal of bone at the interlaminar space to relieve spinal stenosis or nerve root compression.
- **Foraminotomy**: Excision of the spinous process and laminae to level of the pedicle; indicated for spinal stenosis, extensive nerve root compression, or HNP; often combined with fusion.
- **Corpectomy**: Removal of discs above and below an affected spinal segment, with grafting for fusion of the anterior column; indicated for multilevel stenosis or spondylolisthesis (displacement of the anterior column) with nerve root compression; potential post-operative complications include neurologic damage, infection, dural tears, and nonunion.

PHYSICAL THERAPY INTERVENTIONS POST-SPINAL SURGERY

The main goal of physical therapy for patients who have undergone spinal surgery is ambulation. This means that therapy is generally limited to functional mobilization, gait and body mechanics training, proper use of assistive devices, and relaxation and breathing exercises to manage pain. Precautions for spinal surgery patients who have undergone a decompression procedure alone (such as microdiscectomy) can generally lift up to 10 pounds, but those who have also had a spinal fusion or instrumentation inserted should follow the physician's orders for lifting restrictions and should avoid bending and twisting. Logrolling out of bed is recommended for all. Use of rolling walkers is suggested for correct gait, and most patients wear braces out of bed. Special considerations related to specific procedures include use of a splinting pillow and corset in patients whose surgery was done anteriorly; use of ice at the site of iliac crest bone grafting to minimize swelling; and chair sitting as tolerated, if interbody fusion cages were inserted. Cigarette smoking is contraindicated for spinal fusion patients. Patients who have had minimally invasive spine surgeries should be treated similarly.

VERTEBROPLASTY AND KYPHOPLASTY

Vertebroplasty and kyphoplasty are minimally invasive surgeries for progressive osteoporotic vertebral compression fractures, either sudden ones, occurring subsequent to trauma and accompanied by pain and muscle spasm, or anterior wedge compression fractures, in which vertebral height decreases over time with negligible pain. The procedures are inappropriate if there is neurologic damage. In vertebroplasty, polymethylmethacrylate (PMMA) cement is percutaneously injected into the vertebral space for stabilization (but there is no height or deformity restitution). Kyphoplasty is similar, except that the PMMA is more precisely inserted using an inflatable balloon and height deficits and deformities are more likely to be restored because the cement is retained. The main goals of post-surgical physical therapy for each are functional mobility and ambulation. The patient should also be taught good body mechanics, how to log roll for bed transfers, and, if indicated, extremity active range-of-motion and light strengthening exercises.

SOFT-TISSUE REPAIR AND RECONSTRUCTION SURGERIES ON THE KNEE

Most soft-tissue repair and reconstruction surgeries performed on the knee are done arthroscopically, which means the joint is inspected and repaired using a small incision and an endoscope. There are six common types of knee arthroscopy performed. Two involve a meniscus, or cartilage disc, on either the medial or lateral side. A meniscectomy is the complete or partial removal of a meniscus subsequent to an irreparable tear, while a meniscal repair is resolution of a tear in a vascular region of the meniscus, where healing is likely. A lateral retinacular release is the freeing of the synovium, capsular and retinacular structures lateral to the patella, and the proximal muscle fibers of the vastus lateralis. The anterior and posterior cruciate ligaments, which form a cross shape in the knee cap area, are reconstructed if insufficient using anterior cruciate ligament (ACL) or posterior cruciate ligament (PCL) reconstruction. These reconstructions utilize autografts or allografts of the patellar or hamstring tendons (ACL) or the patellar or Achilles tendons (PCL). A quadricepsplasty is a separation and/or lengthening of the quadriceps mechanism. Autologous cartilage transplantation is also being done to repair cartilage.

PHYSICAL THERAPY INTERVENTIONS POST-KNEE REPAIR

The suggested physical therapy for meniscal repair, or meniscectomy, is edema control, proximal and distal range-of-motion (ROM) exercises, functional training per prescribed weight-bearing precautions, and quadriceps and hamstring strengthening, if prescribed. Patients who have had meniscal repair may be instructed to wear a brace or have ROM and weight-bearing restrictions. Physical therapy indications for patients who have had a lateral retinacular release are edema management; gentle ROM and functional training, as prescribed; isometric exercises; and straight-leg raises for quadriceps strengthening. Patients who have had reconstructive surgery on their anterior or posterior cruciate ligaments (ACL or PCL, respectively) should receive edema control, active and passive knee ROM, isometric exercises for the quadriceps and hamstrings, straight leg raises for quadriceps strengthening, and functional training per weight-bearing restrictions. They should also be taught brace use. For those who have undergone a quadricepsplasty, therapy recommendations are limited knee flexion using a hinged brace, ROM, passive knee extension, active/active-assisted exercises for quads and hamstrings, and functional training per weight-bearing precautions.

SOFT TISSUE REPAIR AND RECONSTRUCTION SURGERIES ON THE SHOULDER

Soft-tissue repair and reconstruction surgeries done on the shoulder are usually done arthroscopically, although rotator cuff damage may require open or mini-open repair. There are three main types of shoulder repair. The first is subacromial decompression, or acromioplasty, which is resection of the undersurface of the acromion, a projection on the scapula. Another is a repair of the rotator cuff, a group of muscles and tendons that stabilize the shoulder. For both of these types of repairs, the suggested physical therapy is use of a sling, edema control, pendulum exercises, active and active-assisted shoulder range of motion (ROM), and ROM for the hand, wrist, and elbow. Depending on the scope of repair, patients who have had rotator cuff repairs may be prescribed self-assisted ROM exercises. Another common shoulder surgery is an anterior reconstruction, also called Bankart repair, which is indicated for persistent anterior instability. It consists of a shift of the anterior capsule and/or repair of the labrum (fibrocartilage). Indicated physical therapy includes sling use, if needed; edema control; limited passive ROM; and ROM for the hand, wrist, and elbow. A final common shoulder surgery is to repair a SLAP tear, or an injury to the superior aspect of the labrum within the shoulder joint where the labrum meets the bicep muscle. Surgery involves either removing or repairing the injured portion of the labrum, depending on the individual injury. Physical therapy interventions may be delayed several weeks postoperatively, as the involved arm is generally immobilized (in a sling) during the acute healing phase. When physical therapy is initiated, it progresses from gentle stretching and ROM exercises to strength exercises as the patient tolerates.

Musculoskeletal Physical Therapy Interventions

RANGE OF MOTION EXERCISES

Range of motion (ROM) is the amount of allowable angular motion at a joint between two bones acting as levers. It is correlated to the functional excursion, the distance the attached muscle can shorten to after maximal stretching. ROM exercises are used therapeutically to maintain joint and soft-tissue mobility. There are three basic types of ROM exercises.

- **Passive ROM (PROM)** is movement produced entirely by an external force, such as the therapist, with no voluntary muscle contraction involved. PROM is appropriate in areas where there is acute inflammation or in patients that should not move parts of their body, such as those on bed rest, paralyzed, or in a coma.
- **Active ROM (AROM)** is movement produced by active contraction of the muscles crossing the indicated joint. AROM exercises are indicated for patients able to contract the needed muscles, for aerobic conditioning, and in areas distal to an area immobilized by fracture, etc.
- **Active-assisted ROM (A-AROM)** is a variation of AROM in which the involved muscles are aided by an additional manual or mechanical outside force. A-AROM is useful in patients with weak musculature.

Other types of ROM exercise are self-assisted ROM and continuous passive motion (CPM), the continuous use of a mechanical device.

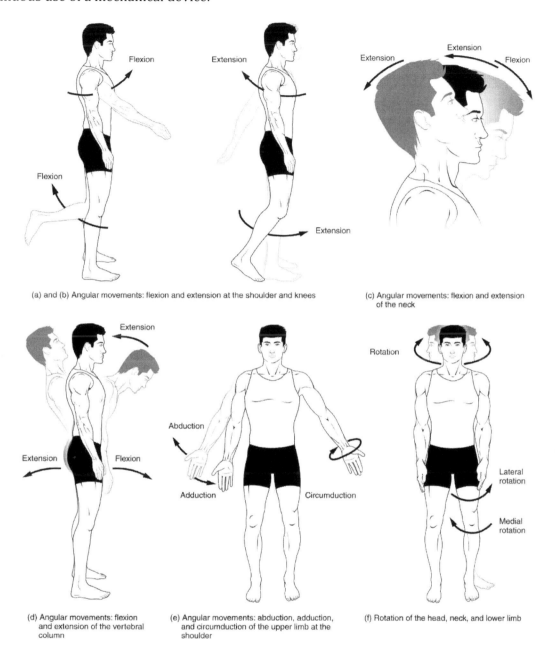

(a) and (b) Angular movements: flexion and extension at the shoulder and knees

(c) Angular movements: flexion and extension of the neck

(d) Angular movements: flexion and extension of the vertebral column

(e) Angular movements: abduction, adduction, and circumduction of the upper limb at the shoulder

(f) Rotation of the head, neck, and lower limb

STRETCHING

Stretching is any type of therapeutic exercise that elongates pathologically shortened soft-tissue structures. The goal is to increase range of motion (ROM). Stretching is indicated anytime ROM is limited due to contractures, adhesions, or scar tissues; in patients with muscle weakness and shortening of opposing tissue; in cases where restricted motion can result in deformities; as part of a fitness program; and before and after exercise to lessen soreness. Stretching is contraindicated with recent fractures, tissue trauma, joint hypermobility, etc. Modes of stretching include:

- **Passive**: Stretching of soft tissue with force applied opposite to direction of muscle shortening.
- **Cyclic**: Repeated passive stretch, generally using a mechanical device.
- **Self-stretching**: Passive stretching of a joint or soft tissue utilizing another body part to apply force.
- **Selective**: Stretching of only certain muscle groups, allowing others to adaptively shorten for functional improvement.
- **Static**: Elongation of soft tissues just past the point of resistance and holding.
- **Ballistic**: High-speed and high-intensity intermittent stretch.
- **Manual**: Force applied by someone else just past resistance.
- **Mechanical**: Use of equipment to produce stretch.
- **Active**: Part of functional movements.
- **Proprioceptive neuromuscular facilitation techniques**

EFFECTIVE STRETCHING INTERVENTIONS

Effective stretching interventions incorporate appropriate use of:

- **Alignment**: The positioning of a limb or the body in a way that allows the stretch force to target the appropriate muscle group.
- **Stabilization**: Securing of one site of attachment of the muscle while force is applied to the other bony attachment.
- **Intensity of stretch**: Magnitude of stretch force applied.
- **Duration of stretch**: Period of time the stretch force is applied during the cycle.
- **Speed of stretch**: How fast the initial stretch force is applied.
- **Frequency of stretch**: Number of stretching periods in a day or week.
- **Mode of stretch**: The manner in which the force is applied, the amount of patient involvement, or the source of the stretch.

ARTHROKINEMATICS

Arthrokinematics describes joint motion in terms of joint shapes, types of joint motion, and other accessory motions. A joint is the connection between two bony partners. The joint shape is either ovoid, where one surface is convex and the other concave, or sellar, in which both surfaces have convex and concave components. Movement of the body lever around the joint is its swing, generally described as flexion, extension, abduction, adduction, or rotation. There are also three potential types of motion between the bony surfaces: rolling of the surface in the same direction as the bony lever movement; sliding (translating) of one surface over the other to a new position, often combined with rolling; or spinning, rotation of one segment about a stationary axis. Other accessory motions include compression, reduction of the space between bony partners; traction, a longitudinal pull; and distraction, separation of bony partners.

JOINT MOBILIZATION

Joint mobilization is the use of manual techniques to control pain and treat joint dysfunctions that reduce range of motion. It addresses specific joint configurations. Joint-play techniques are utilized to reduce pain, muscle guarding, and spasm; reverse joint hypomobility; correct malpositioning or subluxation; treat progressive diseases; and prevent the potential effects of immobility. Prior to use of passive joint mobilization, the patient is examined and evaluated for quality of pain, capsular restriction, and the presence of subluxation or dislocation. There are two possible schemes for grading dosages: graded oscillation techniques and sustained translatory joint-play techniques. The treatment force is applied close to the opposing joint surface either parallel or perpendicular to the treatment plane, such that the entire bone moves and one joint surface glides over the other.

PASSIVE JOINT MOBILIZATION

There are two possible grading systems applied in passive joint mobilization techniques:

- **Graded oscillation techniques**:
  - Grade I: Small rhythmic oscillations at the low end of the available joint play range.
  - Grade II: Large rhythmic oscillations in the available joint play range, not reaching the limit.
  - Grade III: Large rhythmic oscillations performed up to the limit of available joint play and then past it into tissue resistance.
  - Grade IV: Small rhythmic oscillations near the limit of available motion stressed into the tissue resistance range.
  - Grade V: Small-amplitude, high-velocity thrusting method at limit of available motion.
- **Sustained translatory joint play techniques**
  - Grade I (loosening): Small amplitude distraction not involving capsular stress.
  - Grade II (tightening): Application of sufficient distraction or glide to tighten surrounding tissues, involves entire range of available joint play.
  - Grade III (stretching): Larger distraction or glide past tissue resistance, placing stretch on joint capsule and adjacent structures.

MUSCLE PERFORMANCE

Muscle performance is the facility of a muscle to perform work, the amount of energy generated by a force moving through a distance. Muscle performance is related to muscle strength, the force output of a contracting muscle as a function of the amount of tension it can produce; muscle power, the amount of work produced by the muscle per unit of time (force × distance ÷ time); and muscle endurance, the capacity of a muscle to contract repetitively over a long period of time against a load or resistance, while reducing and maintaining tension and resisting fatigue. Two types of training are associated with muscle performance. The first is strength training to develop muscle strength by systematically doing low-repetition or short-duration exercises involving lifting, lowering, or controlling heavy loads. The other is endurance training to improve aerobic power and length of muscle use by doing high-repetition, low-intensity muscle contractions over a prolonged time period. Both are considered resistance exercise or training. Resistance exercise is based on the principle of overload, meaning muscle performance can only improve when the load is above its metabolic capacity.

RESISTIVE TRAINING TERMINOLOGY

Effective resistance training programs incorporate use of appropriate terminology:

- **Alignment**: Proper positioning of patient or body segments
- **Stabilization**: The steadying of proximal or distal joints (on a surface or through body weight) to prevent substitution
- **Intensity**: The amount of load applied
- **Volume**: The product of the total number of repetitions and sets done in a session multiplied by the resistance utilized
- **Exercise order**: The sequence of utilization of muscle groups

- **Frequency**: The number of training periods per day or week
- **Rest interval**: The rest time between exercise sets or sessions
- **Duration**: Total number of weeks or months in the exercise program
- **Mode of exercise**: Definitions provided in terms of type of contraction, weight- or non-weight-bearing position, form of resistance (manual, mechanical, etc.), short- or full-arc range of movement, or energy system involved (anaerobic, aerobic)
- **Velocity**: Speed of exercise
- **Periodization**: The amount of variation
- **Integration of function**: Use of exercises approximating or replicating functional needs

TYPES OF RESISTANCE EXERCISES

The types of resistance exercise are defined in terms of the form of resistance. Broadly speaking, all resistance exercises can be categorized as either manual, meaning the resistance is applied by another person or the individual, or mechanical, involving use of some type of equipment. Resistance exercises can also be differentiated as static, dynamic, isokinetic, or open- or closed-chain. Isometric exercise, in which muscles are under tension and contract but do not change length (such as pushing against a resistance), is a static form of exercise. Dynamic forms of resistance exercise include concentric, in which the muscle shortens while overcoming a load (such as lifting a hand weight), and eccentric, in which less force is used and the muscle fibers lengthen (such as lowering the weight). Isokinetic exercise is also dynamic exercise in which the velocity of limb movement is held constant with a dynamometer but the force is varied. Open- versus closed-chain exercise refers, respectively, to whether the movement is unrestricted or the peripheral segment is restricted with a fixed external resistance.

AQUATIC EXERCISE

Aquatic exercise is the performance of exercises while immersed in a pool or tank of water. Water has buoyancy (an upward force, causing flotation), hydrostatic pressure exerted on immersed objects, viscosity (friction between water molecules), and surface tension. All of these properties make it ideal for performing activities in an environment that is relatively weightless and relaxing, does not put much pressure on joints, acts as a resistance, and keeps certain cardiac parameters in check. Aquatic exercises are means of doing range-of-motion, resistance, weight-bearing, cardiovascular, and functional activity replication exercises. One of the basic principles of aquatic exercise is that fluid in motion adheres to hydromechanics, meaning that slow movement produces parallel or laminar flow, faster movement produces turbulent or non-parallel flow, and turbulence and viscosity together produce drag and increased resistance. Another consideration is thermodynamics, the conversion between forms of energy and the effects of parameters, such as temperature, pressure, and work; for example, with immersion, individuals dissipate less heat. Moreover, the person is governed by a center of buoyancy (at the sternum when vertical) instead of a center of gravity.

Neuromuscular and Nervous Systems

Physical Therapy Data Collection

COMPONENTS OF THE NERVOUS SYSTEM

Structurally, the nervous system consists of the central nervous system (CNS), which includes the brain, cerebellum, brain stem, and spinal cord; and the peripheral nervous system (PNS), which encompasses all parts of the nervous system outside the CNS. The PNS is split into two portions in terms of physiological function: the somatic nervous system, involving sensory organs and responsible for voluntary muscle activity; and the autonomic nervous system (ANS), which controls involuntary bodily processes, such as breathing. Nerve cell types comprising the CNS are neurons and glial cells. Neurons transmit electrochemical impulses. Functionally, they may be afferent, or sensory, neurons, which carry sensory input from peripheral sources through tracts to the CNS; efferent, or motor neurons, that convey messages from the CNS ultimately to peripheral muscles; or interneurons, which link two other neurons. Glial cells do not transmit nerve responses, but they perform important associated functions. They include astrocytes, which are mainly responsible for vascular connections to neurons; oligodendrocytes, which primarily insulate axons (message sending portion of the neuron); and microglia that assist with nervous system repair.

STRUCTURE AND FUNCTIONING OF THE NEURON

A neuron, or nerve cell, is made up of dendrites, extensions that collect information from other neurons; the cell body, comprised of a nucleus and other organelles, where this data is processed; and the axon, a longer extension that transmits impulses to target cells like muscle cells. Most axons are covered with sections of white insulating material made of protein and fats (called myelin sheath) interrupted by unsheathed areas called the nodes of Ranvier. Myelinated axons transmit messages more quickly than unmyelinated ones. Regions of the nervous system, such as the brain and spinal cord, are primarily myelinated and are referred to as white matter. Gray matter, as seen in the part of the brain called the cerebrum, is a highly concentrated area of nerve cell bodies and dendrites. The gap between the axon of one neuron and the dendrite of another is the synapse.

Transmission of information across a synapse is facilitated by chemicals called neurotransmitters, some of the most important being acetylcholine, glutamate, dopamine, and norepinephrine.

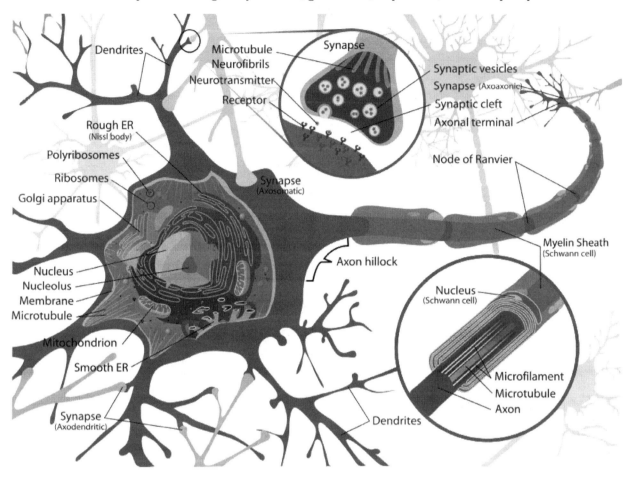

STRUCTURE OF THE CEREBRUM

The cerebrum is the major portion of the brain. It is highly convoluted and covered by gray matter, with white matter internal to that. It consists of four lobes:

- The **frontal lobe** in the front, which controls complex, voluntary motor activities and much of cognitive function.
- The **parietal lobe** behind the frontal lobe, where sensory information is processed and short-term memory resides.

- The **temporal lobe,** centrally located below the frontal and parietal lobes, which performs functions, such as the interpretation of sounds and music, and long-term memory.
- The **occipital lobe** in the back of the head, which is the major visual cortex.

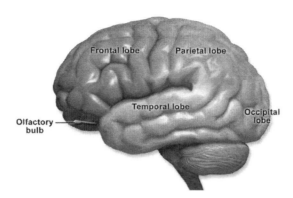

There are association areas, or cortex, between the parietal, temporal, and occipital lobes. The brain, including the cerebrum, has several protective layers, starting with the outer bony skull or cranium. Below that are three membranous layers, or meninges, with spaces between each: the dura mater; the arachnoid; and the pia mater, which is attached to the brain.

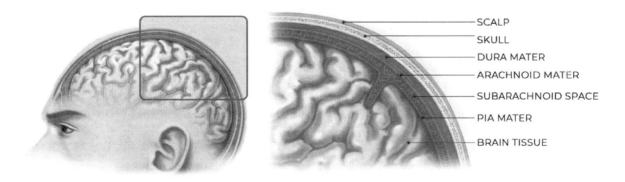

The cerebrum is divided into right and left hemispheres, which are responsible for different functions; neuronal connections between them are called the corpus callosum. There are also deeper brain structures and other brain portions called the cerebellum and brain stem.

SPECIALIZATION OF THE LEFT AND RIGHT CEREBRAL HEMISPHERES

The side of the brain's cerebrum that controls someone's language is deemed the dominant cerebral hemisphere. Ninety-five percent of the populace is left hemisphere dominant, encompassing all right-handed people and about half of left-handed individuals. There are behaviors that have been associated with the left or right hemisphere.

- The **left hemisphere** is the verbal or analytic aspect of the brain. It is associated with behaviors, such as sequential, linear cognitive processing; processing and production of language; reading skills; mathematical computation; sequencing and performance of movements and gestures; and articulation of positive emotions. Damage to the left hemisphere can result in deficits like apraxia (inability to perform complex movements) or lowered speech comprehension.

123

- The **right hemisphere** is linked to nonverbal and artistic abilities. Behaviors associated with the right hemisphere are information processing in a more holistic manner, overall comprehension of concepts, ability to process nonverbal stimuli, visual-spatial perception, mathematical reasoning (as opposed to calculation), posture, sustaining movement, and expression of negative emotions. Right hemisphere damage can lead to poor judgment, irritability, etc.

DEEP SUBCORTICAL STRUCTURES OF THE BRAIN

Deep, subcortical structures in the brain include the internal capsule, the diencephalon, the basal ganglia, and the limbic system:

- The **internal capsule** is the area through which descending fibers from motor areas of the frontal area pass; damage to it can result in contralateral deficits of voluntary movement and ability to perceive touch and positioning.
- The **diencephalon** is quite deep and consists of the thalamus and hypothalamus. It is the zone where the sensory tracts and visual and auditory pathways synapse. The thalamus portion accepts all sensory input (excluding sense of smell) and directs it to the correct cortical area. The hypothalamus lies beneath the thalamus at the base of the brain, and its primary purpose is regulation of homeostasis and autonomic functions.
- The **basal ganglia**, at the base of the cerebrum, regulate motor functions like posture and muscle tone, as well as cognitive functions. Damage to basal ganglia can result in neurological diseases, such as Parkinson's disease and postural instability.
- The **limbic system** runs through various areas of the diencephalon and cortex; its functions are memory-related and include regulation of certain behaviors (sexual interest, pleasure, etc.).

CEREBELLUM AND THE BRAIN STEM

The cerebellum is comprised of two symmetric hemispheres situated below the occipital lobe of the cerebrum of the brain and behind the brain stem. It plays a role in balance and posture maintenance. It also regulates complex muscular movements in a number of ways, including coordinating multi-joint movements, controlling a number of parameters related to muscle contraction, and sequencing of muscle firing during certain movements.

The brain stem is situated between the base of the cerebrum and the spinal cord. It is comprised of three sections with different functions:

- The **midbrain**: At the upper portion; acts as a conduit between the diencephalon and pons; has reflex centers for sight, sound, and touch.
- The **pons**: Below the midbrain; houses axon bundles that connect the cerebellum to other parts of the central nervous system; has functions such as regulation of breathing, orientation of the head, and transmission of facial motor and sensory information (via cranial nerves V to VIII).
- The **medulla**: Below the pons; contains fiber tracts into the spinal cord, which control neck and mouth motor and sensory functions, the heart, and respiratory rate.

The brain stem also contains the reticular activating system, which controls things like the sleep-wake cycle.

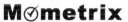

ANATOMY OF THE SPINAL CORD

The spinal cord extends from the medulla in the brain stem, through the vertebral column that protects it, down the level of the initial lumbar vertebra. Starting at the top is the cervical segment, followed by the thoracic segment, the lumbar segment, the sacral segment, and, finally, the dural sac, including the cauda equina (an area of nerve roots for spinal nerves L2 to S5) and the filum terminale connecting to the coccyx. There are 8 cervical nerves, 12 thoracic nerves, 5 lumbar nerves, 5 sacral nerves, and 1 coccygeal nerve. The center of the spinal cord consists of gray matter in a sort of butterfly pattern. The upper dorsal, or posterior horn, of this region transmits sensory stimuli, while the lower ventral, or anterior horn, conveys primarily motor impulses. The outer portion of the spinal cord is white matter, containing tracts of groups of nerve fibers. There are two main afferent (ascending) sensory tracts: the dorsal column, which transmits information about position, vibration, deep touch, and two-point discrimination; and the anterolateral spinothalamic tract, conveying data about light, touch, and pressure. There is one major efferent (descending) motor tract, called the corticospinal tract, which directs skilled movements in extremities, as well as other descending tracts with specific motor functions.

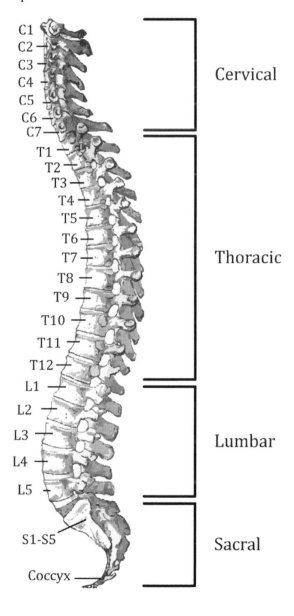

ANTERIOR HORN CELLS, MOTOR UNITS, AND MUSCLE SPINDLES

An anterior horn cell is a larger neuron in the central gray matter of the spinal cord. Its axons ultimately connect to peripheral nerves that innervate muscle fibers. One type of anterior horn cell, called an alpha motor neuron, innervates skeletal. A motor unit is therefore defined as one alpha motor neuron and the muscle fibers it innervates. There are also gamma motor neurons that convey messages to the muscle spindle, which is a sensory organ in skeletal muscle primarily involved with the stretch response and deep tendon reflexes. The muscle spindle is important because it directly transmits sensory input to the spinal cord without the need for higher cortical interpretation.

SOMATIC NERVOUS SYSTEM

The somatic (body) nervous system is the portion of the peripheral nervous system (PNS) that is involved with voluntary reactions to stimuli. It is composed of 12 pairs of cranial nerves, 31 pairs of spinal nerves, and related ganglia and cell bodies. The 12 cranial nerves are situated in the brain stem, and they have various names related to their primary sensory or motor function in the head region (for example, cranial nerve I is olfactory, involved with the sense of smell). Each spinal nerve has a sensory and motor component that comes through an intervertebral foramen between vertebra, where they divide into rami or divisions, beginning the PNS. The uppermost spinal nerves are eight cervical nerves, of which C1 to C4 form the cervical plexus innervating muscles in the neck and shoulder region. The C5 to C8 cervical and T1 thoracic nerve roots comprise the brachial plexus, whose five main nerves innervate most upper-extremity musculature. There are actually 12 thoracic nerves, the rest of which are primarily involved with trunk functions. Lower-extremity muscles are innervated by the nerves forming the lumbosacral plexus, the five lumbar (L1 to L5) and first three (S1 to S3) of five sacral nerves. Peripheral nerves connect to the system efferently, eventually innervating motor end plates in muscles; or afferently, originating in the skin, muscle tendon, or Golgi tendon organ.

AUTONOMIC NERVOUS SYSTEM

The autonomic nervous system (ANS) is the portion of the peripheral nervous system involved with regulation of involuntary functions, such as respiration and metabolism. Control centers for the ANS are situated in the hypothalamus and brain stem, and regulation within the system is achieved through a two-way pathway between the central nervous system and organs. The ANS is comprised of two types of nerve fibers: sympathetic nerve fibers that originate in the thoracic and upper lumbar parts of the spinal cord and regulate functions in the abdominal region affected by stress, such as heart rate, blood pressure, and temperature; and parasympathetic fibers responsible for homeostasis or maintenance of fundamental bodily functions. Parasympathetic responses are derived from cranial nerves III, VII, IX, and X in the brain stem (X being the important vagus nerve, which innervates the myocardium and lung and digestive tract smooth muscles) and sacral nerves S2 to S5, which regulate bowel, bladder, and external genitalia functions. The primary neurotransmitters involved are norepinephrine and acetylcholine for sympathetic and parasympathetic divisions, respectively.

BLOOD CIRCULATION AND NERVOUS SYSTEM FUNCTION

Neurons within the brain must receive an adequate blood supply constantly as they are incapable of performing glycolysis (the breakdown of carbohydrates to produce energy) or storing glycogen. Most of the cerebrum is supplied with blood through the carotid and cerebral arteries, which ascend originally from the aortic arch anteriorly. The brain stem and part of the occipital and temporal lobes are supplied blood via the basilar artery and its branches, which are other cerebral arteries. A protective mechanism that alleviates the potential danger of blood vessel occlusion in

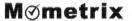

the brain is the circle of Willis at its base, where the basilar artery and several carotid and cerebral arteries are interconnected.

CAUSES OF NERVE CELL DAMAGE

Neurons in any portion of the nervous system that are denied oxygen cannot regenerate and, thus, die. They also release excess glutamate, which can damage neighboring nerve cells. Nerve cell death usually occurs in the central nervous system within minutes of artery obstruction. Typically, within a day or so, the necrotic tissue liquefies and forms a cyst and then a glial scar. Within four or five days, adjoining healthy axons move in to form compensating networks. Peripheral nerve injuries are not usually due to obstruction but rather situations like stretching, compression, or disease. Therefore, the compensatory mechanism is typically different. Here, basically, there is axonal necrosis distal to the site, separation from the myelin sheath, phagocytosis by Schwann cells, and wallerian degeneration of postsynaptic cells. If the peripheral nerve injury is minimal involving only the axon, regeneration may occur through sprouting at the proximal end and the corresponding muscle may eventually be re-innervated.

MOTOR CONTROL

Motor control is the capacity to sustain and change posture and movement. It involves both the neurologic and muscular systems. It is an interaction between the individual, the task at hand, and the surrounding environment. Motor control utilized for specific tasks is a function of the person's cognitive and perceptual status, which can change over time. Motor control must be utilized within milliseconds to be functional, making deficits potentially dangerous. Sensory stimuli can elicit reflexive motor responses, and there are higher levels of motor control, the utmost being voluntary movement.

HIERARCHIC THEORY OF MOTOR CONTROL

The hierarchic theory of motor control states that the cortex of the brain exerts ultimate control over motor functions, the development of certain motor behaviors in childhood is related to maturation of the brain, the highest stage of motor control is the ability to perform voluntary movement, and reflexes are the basic motor control units. It defines a reflex as the coupling of a sensory stimulus and motor response, which for simple reflexes requires only three neurons: the sensory neuron and the associated interneuron and motor neuron derived from the spinal cord. There are also higher-level tonic reflexes, affecting muscle tone and posture and involving the brain stem, and complex postural responses, associated with the midbrain and cortex, such as righting reactions, equilibrium reactions, and protective reactions in extremities.

STAGES OF MOTOR CONTROL AND POSTURAL CONTROL

According to hierarchal theory, infants go through four stages of motor control: mobility, random movement during approximately the first three months of life; stability or static postural, the capacity to maintain a stable, weight-bearing, antigravity posture; controlled mobility (also known as dynamic postural control), mobility combined with postural stability; and skilled movement patterns, such as reaching or walking. There are two types of stability: tonic holding, which is mainly isometric (for example, prone extension); and co-contraction, which involves static contraction of antagonistic muscles at a joint for stability. Co-contraction is the mechanism invoked for various prone positions, a semi-squat, and standing. Combined with weight shifting or movement to another position, co-contraction becomes controlled mobility. Postural control, the capacity to maintain body alignment and balance, develops sequentially, as well, in the following order: righting reactions, head and trunk movements facilitating orientation or alignment; protective reactions, extremity movements in response to displacement, such as moving a limb to prepare for falling; and equilibrium reactions, counteracting responses that maintain the center of gravity within a base of support.

SYSTEMS MODELS OF MOTOR CONTROL

There are various systems models of motor control. Some of the basic tenets of each are that:

- Motor control is a complex interaction between a number of bodily systems, including the nervous, musculoskeletal, and cardiopulmonary systems, and posture.
- Posture and movement occur in a logical fashion.
- Movement control is either dependent on past success through feedback (a closed-loop model) or a cued, preprogrammed response (open-loop model).

Postural control, the correlation between posture and movement, is essential to motor control in these models. Further, there are seven components to postural control: staying within the limits of stability, which means having the center of gravity within one's base of support; adaptation of posture to the current environment; functioning musculoskeletal and neurologic systems; a predictive central set (anticipatory postural readiness); muscular coordination or timely sequencing; stabilization of the eyes and head; and sensory organization. Sensory organization, in terms of posture and balance, means use of functioning visual, vestibular (balance-related functions initiated in the ear), and somatosensory (touch, proprioception) systems.

NASHNER'S MODEL OF POSTURAL CONTROL

Nashner's model of postural control is a paradigm for control of standing balance. It posits that there are three sway strategies that allow balanced standing. In adults, the first is the ankle strategy, in which the person sways from the ankles, always coming back to midline through use of the anterior tibialis and gastrocnemius muscles. Another is the hip strategy, where the individual sways from the hips, activating in sequence proximal to distal muscles. This strategy is useful on narrow bases of support, such as balance beams. The last is the stepping strategy, where the person steps while swaying. Some children employ the ankle sway strategy as early as 18 months and occasionally the hip strategy, but the expected use of sway strategies as quickly as adults occurs at 7-10 years of age.

MOTOR LEARNING

Motor learning is the process by which a lasting change in motor performance occurs through practice or experience. For infants, motor learning involves the perfection of certain tasks, such as learning to walk. For any given individual, the time it takes to learn a specific motor task is contingent on the task's difficulty, the person's motivation to learn it, the amount of practice completed, and the amount of feedback received. People go through three phases of motor learning before perfecting a new task.

- The first is the **cognitive phase**, where the individual uses sensory input, such as verbal directions and vision, to figure out what the task involves. This stage requires a high degree of attention to the task at hand and is difficult for patients who have undergone brain injuries or cerebrovascular accidents.
- The second period is a longer **associative phase**, in which the individual makes a number of trials and uses sensory feedback to get better with time by detecting errors and correcting them.
- The last stage is the **autonomous phase**, where the task has been mastered and can be completed with little attention to it and minimal sensory input.

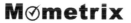

THEORIES OF MOTOR LEARNING

Prevalent theories of motor learning include:

- **Adams' closed-loop theory** posits that intrinsic (internally derived) feedback and extrinsic feedback (knowledge of results) are used to develop the correct feel of new movements. It explains how slow movements might be learned but not faster ones.
- **Schmidt's schema theory** says that once a motor program, or a learned motor task, is developed, it can be recalled with minimal cognitive or cortical input because muscle commands are preprogrammed unless parameters change. Further, it expounds that feedback during movement can be derived from the muscles as they contract during the movement, the portions of the body that are moving, and/or the surrounding environment. Thus, learned actions are under both open-loop and closed-loop control. These assumptions explain learning of both slow and fast movements.

HUMAN DEVELOPMENT

LIFESPAN APPROACH TO DEVELOPMENT

Developmental change throughout life can be viewed in a number of ways. These views include a triangular view, with development peaking during maturity and declining with age; a plateau view, which is similar, except maturity is more prolonged; a continuous circle or life-cycle view, where the beginning and end are similar; or as multidimensional and intertwined. The latter view is consistent with the lifespan approach to development as espoused by Bates, which says that development has five characteristics; it is life-long; multidimensional; plastic and flexible; contextual; and entrenched in history. Thus, a lifespan view of motor development regards change as a continual process from conception to death.

DEVELOPMENTAL TIME PERIODS

The developmental time periods can be broken down into the following phases:

- The first developmental time period is **infancy**, defined as birth to two years of age, when sensory data is used to cue movement and explore the environment.
- **Childhood** spans from age two years to the time of adolescence, which differs for girls (age 10) and boys (age 12). Childhood is the time period when an individual learns movement strategies and solutions for daily problems, primarily centered around themselves with parental help during early childhood and more interactive and concrete later.
- **Adolescence** is defined as the time directly proceeding and continuing into and after puberty, which is roughly 10-18 years of age for females and 12-20 years of age for males. It is a period of intense physical and emotional changes, including establishment of individual identity, formation of values, development of vocational aspirations, and development of the ability to solve abstract problems.
- Adolescents slowly transition into **early adulthood**, which starts approximately at age 18 for females and 20 for males and extends to age 40.
- **Middle and older adulthood** have been defined as from 40-65 years and from 65 years to death, respectively. Older adulthood has been further divided into the young-old (65-74 years), middle-old (75-84 years), and old-old (85 years or older).

PIAGET'S THEORY OF COGNITIVE DEVELOPMENT

Piaget believed that development was progressive and followed a set pattern. He believed the child's environment, their interactions with others in that environment, and how the environment responds help to shape their cognitive development. There are **4 stages to Piaget's theory:**

- The **sensorimotor stage (birth to age 2)** is when the child learns to work toward a goal, the relationship between cause and effect, that objects still exist even though they cannot see them, and a sense of self.
- In the **preoperational stage (ages 2-7)** language skills develop, the child only sees their own point of view, they do not think abstractly, and have a difficult time telling fact from fantasy.
- The **concrete operations stage (ages 7-11)** is when children begin to understand relationships between objects and events, learn to classify and use patterns, understand that some occurrences are reversible, and see other's points of view.
- The **formal operations stage (ages 12 years and older)** is the stage of abstract thinking, better reasoning skills, and forward thinking.

MASLOW'S HIERARCHY OF NEEDS

Maslow defined human motivation in terms of needs and wants. His **hierarchy of needs** is classically portrayed as a pyramid sitting on its base divided into horizontal layers. He theorized that, as humans fulfill the needs of one layer, their motivation turns to the layer above. The layers consist of (from bottom to top):

- **Physiological**: The need for air, fluid, food, shelter, warmth, and sleep.
- **Safety**: A safe place to live, a steady job, a society with rules and laws, protection from harm, and insurance or savings for the future.
- **Love/Belonging**: A network consisting of a significant other, family, friends, co-workers, religion, and community.
- **Esteem or self-respect**: The knowledge that you are a person who is successful and worthy of esteem, attention, status, and admiration.
- **Self-actualization**: The acceptance of your life, choices, and situation in life and the empathetic acceptance of others, as well as the feeling of independence and the joy of being able to express yourself freely and competently.

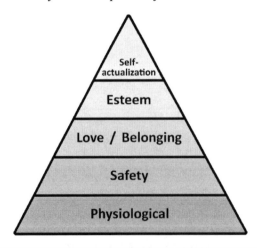

Review Video: **Maslow's Hierarchy of Needs**
Visit mometrix.com/academy and enter code: 461825

ERIKSON'S DEVELOPMENTAL TASKS

The developmental tasks according to Erik Erikson:

- **Trust vs. Mistrust (Birth to 1 year)**: Trust, faith and optimism develop if the needs of warmth, food and love are met. If not, this can result in mistrust.
- **Autonomy vs. Shame/Doubt (Ages 1-3)**: The child desires independence in basic self-care tasks and wants choice. If independence is not encouraged, this can lead to doubt and shame. Independence develops self-control and willpower.
- **Initiative vs. Guilt (Ages 3-6)**: The child engages in self-directed play and starts activities without outside influence. Imaginative play and competition are introduced. This can lead to guilt or direction and purpose based on how this initiative is supportive.
- **Industry vs. Inferiority (Ages 6-12)**: The child values feeling capable and competent, and develops a sense of pride and self-worth. They desire to do what is right and good. Social interactions between peers becomes more important, and comparing achievements can result in feelings of pride or feelings of inferiority if not properly guided.
- **Identity vs. Role Confusion (Ages 12-18)**: Parents, teachers, peers, family members, church, culture, and ethnicity all role model and pressure youth to adopt certain behaviors. The task of adolescents is to discover their own identity.
- **Intimacy vs. Isolation (Ages 18-40)**: Young people learn to commit to another person in a love or family relationship. They learn the behavior required to maintain this relationship.
- **Generativity vs. Stagnation (Ages 40-65)**: Adults have many tasks when they try to find their own interests and niche in the work world. Family, community, and work roles are defined.
- **Integrity vs. Despair (Ages 65+)**: Older people ponder their life experiences to put them into perspective. They learn to accept the aging process and begin to think about their own death.

COMMON DEVELOPMENTAL CONCEPTS

All developmental concepts embrace the notion that motor development is epigenetic, meaning it develops through successive gradual changes, and that there is a series of gross-motor milestones children pass. There are two types of concepts regarding development:

- **Directional concepts** include: cephalocaudal development, the idea that head movements are mastered before trunk ones; proximal to distal, meaning that an infant works to establish midline control in the head and neck before shoulders, pelvis, and extremities; mass to specific movements, in other words mastering whole body movements before isolated or dissociated ones; and gross to fine, proceeding from large muscle to more discreet movements.
- **Kinesiologic concepts** are based upon the observation that shortly after birth, infants are in physiologic flexion, meaning their limbs and trunk are naturally in a flexed position. Only over time do they move toward antigravity extension and later antigravity flexion, then lateral flexion, and, ultimately, rotation.

PROCESSES INVOLVED IN DEVELOPMENT

The three processes involved in development are growth, maturation, and adaptation:

- **Growth** is defined as any expansion in dimension or proportion, usually quantified in terms of parameters like height, weight, and head circumference.
- **Maturation** is the full development of certain internal body processes as genetically programmed, such as internal organs becoming more complex or the emergence of secondary sexual characteristics.
- **Adaptation** is the course by which physical changes occur in response to environmental stimuli, such as the way in which musculoskeletal strength is developed through performance of functional activities.

GROSS AND FINE MOTOR MILESTONES IN INFANTS

Gross- and fine-motor milestones refer to expected developmental milestones involving large movements and small muscle movements, respectively.

- The **expected gross-motor milestones** are head control by 4 months; log rolling followed by segmental rolling, achieved by 6-8 months; independent sitting by 8 months; cruising (walking sideways using hands or tummy) by 9 months; reciprocal creeping by 10 months; and walking by age 12 months (range 7-18 months).
- The **expected fine-motor milestones** of development include a palmar grasp reflex present at birth; hand awareness or regard at 2 months; raking at 5 months; and development of a voluntary palmar grasp by age 6 months. This voluntary grasp should develop further over the next few months to become radial palmar (adduction of thumb) at 7 months; radial digital (use of fingers as well) by 9 months; use of thumb with index finger in various arrangements (inferior and superior pincher) by 12 months; and a three-jaw chuck grasp in the same time period. Infants should be able to release a grasped object voluntarily at about 7-9 months, with further control developed within the next few months.

STAGES OF INFANT DEVELOPMENT THROUGH 10 MONTHS OF AGE

During the first two months of life, the infants' internal body processes stabilize, essential biologic rhythms are developed, and they can spontaneously grasp and release and do unilateral head lifting on all fours. At ages 3-4 months, infants have developed forearm support, head control, and midline orientation. This enables them to do things such as support themselves while prone on their elbows, perform primitive rolling without rotation, and hold their head upright while being held vertical or tilted. At 4-5 months, they start to gain antigravity control of the extensors and flexors, and they can do bottom lifting and dissociate head and limb movements. They often assume a posture that looks like swimming. By 6 months, the infant has strong extension-abduction of the extremities and complete extension of the trunk. They pivot in a circle on their tummy and right themselves using the Landau reflex, can do segmental rolling (essential for transitions), can sit up if placed and supported, can be pulled up to sitting or standing, and can do some reaching. By 7-8 months, their trunk control has developed to the point that they can do balanced sitting, have some spontaneous trunk rotation, and can ambulate via pre-walking mechanisms like belly crawling. By ages 9-10 months, movement progresses to crawling, creeping, pulling themselves up to stand, and cruising.

TODDLER DEVELOPMENT

A toddler is a young child learning to walk, the phase generally defined as starting at age 1 year and extending through age 2. By 12 months of age, the infants typically try slow independent walking

132

using their hands for guarding. Their skill at walking usually progresses by age 16-17 months to the point where they can carry or pull objects at the same time, walk sideways and backwards, and navigate stairs one step at a time. They have learned to rise from supine to standing through rolling, four-point prone, plant grade, squat, and semi-squat positions. Most toddlers demonstrate adult gait characteristics, such as reciprocal arm swing and heel strike by 18 months. They should be able to squat easily and pick up toys by age 20-22 months and ambulate quickly with arm swing closely approximating an adult by age 24 months. Older toddlers can do easy types of jumps, typically done from one foot landing on the other at 18 months, jumping up from and landing with two feet at 24 months, and progressing to increasingly more difficult types.

MOVEMENT PATTERNS DEVELOPED FROM AGES 3-6 YEARS

The majority of experts concur that most children achieve a mature gait pattern by age 3 years and almost all do by age 4. Three-year-olds can also accomplish other reciprocal activities, such as climbing a ladder and more difficult jumps than before. Children acquire good enough static and dynamic balance by age 4 to do things like prolonged one-foot standing, sequential hopping, galloping, and catching a ball. These skills are developed further by age 5, when they also encompass things such as skipping on alternating feet and kicking. Hand dominance, the regular use of one hand over the other for tasks like throwing or eating, is established by this time period. Balance and coordination are further developed by age 6, and the child can master other forms of locomotion like bike riding. Adult approximations of activities, such as running, are possible in the 6-to-10-year age range. Movement patterns, while generally established by age 10, can be changed at later ages into adulthood. In older individuals, these pattern changes are often related to pathological changes, such as stiffening of joints; these persons often revert to a more asymmetrical pattern as seen in young children, rather than the symmetrical patterns typical from adolescence through adulthood.

POSTURAL CHANGES ASSOCIATED WITH AGING FROM INFANCY TO CHILDHOOD

When babies are born, they have a forward flexed curve in the thoracic region and another in the sacral region. As they proceed through infancy and learn movements, convex forward cervical and lumbar curves also develop. When viewed laterally, a young person in standing posture has a vertical gravity line that goes linearly at a right angle to the ground through the middle of the earlobe, the middle of the acromion process of the shoulder, the greater trochanter of the hip, the knee behind the patella but in front of the joint, and a point slightly in front of the lateral malleolus of the ankle. Essentially posture is quite straight. However, as we age, the secondary spinal curves tend to decrease, intervertebral discs often stiffen and flatten, and other changes may occur as a result of a sedentary lifestyle or prolonged sitting. The typical standing posture of an older person is more forward and less straight than that of a younger person. This may be accompanied by demineralization of bone, decreased flexibility at the joints, loss of strength, and changes in gait and balance.

BALANCE AND GAIT CHANGES ASSOCIATED WITH AGING

Older adults may have significant problems related to balance and falling. Many of these problems are associated with neurologic changes. Sensory receptors involved with positioning, head movement, awareness of vibration, or vision are often changed structurally by this point, thus reducing the quality of information received. In addition, musculoskeletal changes, such as loss of some joint range of motion and muscular strength, make it more difficult to respond quickly and establish balance. Gait changes associated with aging include decreased cadence and stride length and use of a wider base of support for increased balance.

NEUROLOGIC DATA COLLECTION

Data collection for the neurological system includes:

- Assess the **health history** for any trauma, falls, alcoholism, drug abuse, medications taken, and family history of neurological problems.
- Ask about any presenting **neurological symptoms**, the circumstances in which they occur, whether they fluctuate, and any associated factors, such as seizures, pain, vertigo, weakness, abnormal sensations, visual problems, loss of consciousness, changes in cognition, and motor problems.

Data collection also includes determining the level of consciousness and cognition. Posture and movements are observed for abnormalities. Facial expression and movement are noted. Cranial nerve assessment is done. The patient is assessed for strength, coordination, and balance and the ability to perform ADLs. One should assess for clonus and test all reflexes, including Babinski, gag, blink, swallow, upper and lower abdominal, cremasteric in males, plantar, perianal, biceps, triceps, brachioradialis, patellar and ankle. Peripheral sensation is tested by touching the patient with cotton balls and the sharp and dull ends of a broken tongue blade.

> **Review Video: Nervous System**
> Visit mometrix.com/academy and enter code: 708428

DESCRIBING LEVELS OF CONSCIOUSNESS

Level of consciousness is an indication of a person's mental status and is potentially predictive of severity and prognosis. A normal awake, attentive, interactive level of consciousness is described as **alert**. A person who needs various increasing levels of arousal and experiences increasing states of confusion can be described in order as **lethargic, obtunded**, or in stupor (semi-coma). A patient who cannot be aroused and may have missing reflex responses is defined as being in a **coma** or deep coma. Other abnormal states of consciousness include **delirium**, disorientation accompanied by irritation, misperception, and offensive behavior, and **dementia**, an altered mental state due to organic disease but not involving altered arousal.

GLASGOW COMA SCALE

The Glasgow coma scale (GCS) measures the depth and duration of coma or impaired level of consciousness and is used for postoperative assessment by the health care team. The physical therapist assistant must be familiar with the GCS scoring system to understand the status of their patient. The GCS measures three parameters: best eye response, best verbal response, and best motor response, with a total possible score that ranges from 3 to 15:

Eye opening	4: Spontaneous 3: To verbal stimuli 2: To pain (not of face) 1: No response
Verbal	5: Oriented 4: Conversation confused, but can answer questions 3: Uses inappropriate words 2: Speech incomprehensible 1: No response

Motor	6: Moves on command
	5: Moves purposefully respond pain
	4: Withdraws in response to pain
	3: Decorticate posturing (flexion) in response to pain
	2: Decerebrate posturing (extension) in response to pain
	1: No response

Injuries/conditions are classified according to the total score: 3-8 Coma; ≤8 Severe head injury likely requiring intubation; 9-12 Moderate head injury; 13-15 Mild head injury.

> **Review Video: Glasgow Coma Scale**
> Visit mometrix.com/academy and enter code: 133399

RANCHOS LOS AMIGOS SCALE OF COGNITIVE FUNCTIONING

The Rancho Los Amigos Scale of Cognitive Functioning describes levels of cognitive functioning. It is useful for evaluating traumatic brain injury and other patients with various levels of cognitive ability. There are 10 levels. Characteristic behavior is described for each. Patients at levels I, II, and III (No Response, Generalized Response, Localized Response, respectively) require total assistance. Those at levels IV (Confused/Agitated) and V (Confused, Inappropriate, Nonagitated) require maximal assistance. A level VI patient is Confused, Appropriate, needing moderate assistance; and one at level VII is Automatic, Appropriate, needing minimal assistance for performance of daily living skills. Levels VIII and IX (both Purposeful, Appropriate) necessitate only standby assistance, the latter upon request; an individual at level X is also Purposeful, Appropriate, but independent with modifications.

MENTAL STATUS EXAM

Appropriate cognitive functions to evaluate during a mental status examination are attention, orientation, memory, calculation, construction, abstraction, and judgment:

- **Attention**, the ability to mentally focus on a stimulus or task, can be tested by asking patients to repeat series of numbers or letters or spell words.
- **Orientation**, the facility to understand in terms of person, place, and time, can be assessed by asking patients questions such as their name, age, address, etc.
- **Memory** has three components: immediate recall, short-term memory, and long-term memory, which can each be addressed by asking patients to recount words after a few seconds, words after a few minutes, or past events.
- **Calculation** is the ability to solve mathematical problems, which can be assessed by asking them to perform simple calculations involving whole numbers.
- **Construction** is the capacity to construct a multidimensional shape, which can be tested by having patients draw a figure.
- **Abstraction** is the capacity for abstract as opposed to literal reasoning, which can be assessed with object comparison.
- **Judgment** is the ability to reason, which can be determined by having patients demonstrate common sense and safety.

CRANIAL NERVE ASSESSMENT

The cranial nerves and their accompanying function and test are as follows:

	Name	Function	Test
I	Olfactory	Smell	Test olfaction
II	Optic	Visual acuity	Snellen eye chart; Accommodation
III	Oculomotor	Eye movement/ pupil	Pupillary reflex; Eye/eyelid motion
IV	Trochlear	Eye movement	Eye moves down & out
V	Trigeminal	Facial motor/ sensory	Corneal reflex; Facial sensation; Mastication
VI	Abducens	Eye movement	Lateral eye motion
VII	Facial	Facial expression; Taste	Moves forehead, closes eyes, smile/frown, puffs cheeks; Taste
VIII	Vestibulocochlear (Acoustic)	Hearing; Balance	Hearing (Weber/Rinne tests); Nystagmus
IX	Glossopharyngeal	Pharynx motor/sensory	Gag reflex; Soft palate elevation
X	Vagus	Visceral sensory, motor	Gag, swallow, cough
XI	Accessory	Sternocleidomastoid and trapezius (motor)	Turns head & shrugs shoulders against resistance
XII	Hypoglossal	Tongue movement	Push out tongue; move tongue from side to side

VISION TESTING

Vision testing as part of a neurologic examination should include cranial nerve testing and further examination of the pupils by the physician for size and similarity, shape, and reactivity. Normally, the pupils of both eyes should be the same size (maximal 1 mm difference) and that size should be 2-4 mm in light and 4-8 mm in darkness. Normal pupils are round, but if the person has neurologic dysfunction, they may appear oval or irregular. Reactivity is tested by shining a light into the eye, which normally constricts the pupil but produces no or some other type of reaction in people with neurologic conditions. On the other hand, moving into darkness should normally dilate the pupils. The clinician also observes for nystagmus, involuntary rhythmic movement of the eyes, which can indicate equilibrium problems; cerebellar lesions; or disparity between reflexes coordinating the two eyes. During transfers or ambulation, the therapist can help patients with nystagmus by having them focus on a point or object in front of them.

MOTOR FUNCTION DATA COLLECTION

STRENGTH TESTING

Strength testing is part of the motor function data collection process. Strength is broadly defined as the force output of a contracting muscle, which is a function of the amount of tension it can produce. There are different ways of evaluating strength. Muscle strength can be graded from 0 to 5 or 0 to N (normal) using manual muscle testing, strong or weak when describing ability to do resisted isometrics, or in terms of proportion of available range of motion. Functional strength, the ability of the neuromuscular system to control functional activities in a smooth and coordinated manner, is another way to grade strength.

MUSCLE TONE TESTING

Changes in muscle tone are related to the presence of neurologic lesions or other factors, such as stress, pain, medications, and arousal of the central nervous system. The common abnormalities are:

- **Hypertonicity**, or increased muscle contractility, possibly accompanied by spasticity or rigidity
- **Hypotonicity**, or decreased muscle contractility, usually with flaccidity (less muscle resistance)
- **Dystonia**, disordered tone with involuntary movements.

There are various ways of grading abnormal muscle tone. It can be rated passively as mild, moderate, or severe in terms of resistance; actively in terms of whether the person can perform functional mobility and voluntary movement; or either way as in whether or not they can achieve full range of motion. The Modified Ashworth Scale is a numeric grading system for abnormal tone that rates it from 0 (no increase in muscle tone) to 4 (affected parts are rigid for extension and flexion). For a neurologic exam, a good method is whether the patient has abnormal decorticate (flexion) posturing indicative of corticospinal tract lesions and/or abnormal decerebrate (extension) posturing indicative of brain stem lesions.

REFLEX TESTING

DEEP TENDON REFLEX TESTING

Reflexes are tested if there is suspected neurological involvement associated with musculoskeletal pain. Deep tendon reflexes are investigated by placing the patient in a relaxed supine or sitting position, with the tendon to be tested in a slight stretch, and then striking the tendon with a reflex hammer to see whether a normal response occurs. Deep tendon reflexes are **graded** from 0 to 4 as follows:

- 0: Absent, areflexia
- 1: Diminished, hyporeflexia
- 2: Average, normal
- 3: Exaggerated, brisk
- 4: Clonus, very brisk/hyperreflexia

Each reflex is tested five or six times to see whether the reflex response diminishes, which indicates nerve root issues. Responses can be enhanced using the Jendrassik maneuver (clenching teeth, squeezing hands) when testing the lower limbs or squeezing the legs during upper limb testing.

COMMON DEEP REFLEXES TESTED

Beginning at the top, the common deep tendon reflexes tested and the corresponding central nervous system segments are:

- **Jaw**: C5
- **Biceps**: C5 to C6
- **Brachioradialis**: C5 to C6
- **Triceps**: C7 to C8
- **Patella**: L3 to L4

Tendons are tested to elicit the following reflexes:

- **Tibialis biceps tendon**: To elicit contraction
- **Brachioradialis tendon**: To get elbow flexion and/or forearm pronation
- **Distal triceps tendon**: To trigger elbow extension and muscle contraction
- **Patellar tendon**: For leg extension
- **Tibialis posterior tendon**: To get plantar flexion of the foot with inversion
- **Semimembranosus tendon and biceps femoris tendon**: To elicit knee flexion and muscle contraction
- **Achilles' tendon**: For plantar flexion

SUPERFICIAL REFLEXES

Superficial reflexes are triggered by superficial stroking of a skin area with an object that is sharp but will not break the skin. Common superficial reflexes tested include the upper and lower abdominal, cremasteric, plantar, gluteal, and anal areas. The normal expected responses and the relevant central nervous system segments for each are:

- **Upper abdominal reflex**: Should move the umbilicus up and toward the area being stroked; T7 to T9
- **Lower abdominal reflex**: Should shift the umbilicus down and toward the area being stroked; T11 to T12
- **Cremasteric reflex on the upper, inner part of the male's thigh**: Should elevate the scrotum; T12, L1
- **Plantar reflex on the lateral side of the sole of the foot**: Should produce flexion of toes; S1 to S2
- **Gluteal reflex**: Should tense the skin in that buttock region; L4 to L5, S1 to S3
- **Anal reflex**: Should contract the anal sphincter muscles; S2 to S4

Other superficial reflexes commonly evaluated as part of cranial nerve (CN) testing are corneal, gag, and swallowing.

PATHOLOGICAL REFLEXES

Four reflexes elicit the same response and are associated pathologically with pyramidal tract nervous system lesions. They are as follows:

- **Babinski reflex**, stroking of the lateral aspect of the sole of the foot
- **Chaddock's reflex**, stroking of the lateral side of the foot under the lateral malleolus
- **Oppenheim's reflex**, stroking of the anteromedial tibial surface
- **Gordon's reflex**, firm squeezing of the calf muscles.

These trigger extension of the big toe and fanning of the four small toes if there are pathological lesions. The Babinski is a normal response in newborns and can be indicative of organic hemiplegia. **Hoffman's reflex**, elicited by flicking the end of the index, middle, or ring fingers, will cause the thumb or other non-flicked finger to flex, indicating tetany or pyramidal tract lesions.

Other pathological reflexes involving the lower limbs include the following:

- **Piotrowski's reflex**, dorsiflexion and supination of the foot upon percussion of the tibialis anterior muscle, seen with organic CNS disease.
- **Brudzinski's reflex**, flexion of the other leg upon passive flexion of one leg, suggesting meningitis.

- **Rossolimo's reflex**, flexion of toes when their plantar surface is tapped, indicating pyramidal tract lesions.
- **Schaeffer's reflex**, flexion of toes and foot after pinching the center of the Achilles tendon, indicative of organic hemiplegic.

DERMATOMES, NERVE ROOTS, MYOTOMES, AND SCLEROTOMES

A **dermatome** is a section of skin supplied by a single nerve root of the spine. Peripheral nerves are generally supplied by more than one nerve root and do not necessarily correspond to a single nerve root. A nerve root is the section of the spine from which innervation originates. Beginning at the skull going down, there are eight cervical (C1 to C8), 12 thoracic (T1 to T12), five lumbar (L1 to L5), and four sacral (S1 to S4) nerve roots.

A **myotome** is a group of muscles whose initial innervation is a single nerve root. Injury to a single nerve root causes only incomplete paralysis of the muscles in the myotome, whereas a lesion in a peripheral nerve causes complete paralysis of the associated muscles.

A **sclerotome** is a bone or connective tissue region supplied by a single nerve root.

The significance of dermatomes, myotomes, and sclerotomes is the differentiation between referred and localized pain. This is important in terms of musculoskeletal pain because it is often referred pain.

UPPER QUARTER SCREEN

Upper- and lower-quarter screens are short evaluations for bilateral range of motion, muscle strength, sensations, and deep tendon reflexes. An upper-quarter screen is the evaluation of one side down to generally the T1 nerve root, roughly equivalent to an upper limb scan. For lesions in each nerve root in this area, the following might be observed in the respective myotomes and dermatomes:

Nerve Root	Myotome	Dermatome
C1	Cervical rotation	Vertex of skull
C2	Shoulder shrug	Posterior head
C3	Shoulder shrug	Neck
C4	Shoulder shrug	Acromioclavicular joint
C5	Shoulder abduction	Lateral arm
C6	Wrist extension	Lateral forearm
C7	Elbow extension	Palmar distal phalanx of triceps
C8	Thumb extension	Palmar distal part of triceps
T1	Finger abduction	Medial forearm

This list does not thoroughly examine all possibilities.

LOWER-QUARTER SCREENING

A lower-quarter screening is roughly equivalent to a lower limb scan and involves evaluation on one side from nerve roots L1 to S1or lower. Most thoracic nerve root involvement is hard to localize. For lesions in each nerve root in this area, the following might be observed in the respective myotomes and dermatomes:

Nerve Root	Myotome	Dermatome
L1	Hip flexion	Back and thigh near groin
L2	Hip flexion	Back and front of thigh to knee
L3	Knee extension	Middle third of front thigh
L4	Knee extension	Patella, medial malleolus
L5	Great toe extension	Fibular head, dorsum of foot
S1	Ankle plantar flexion	Lateral malleolus, plantar surface

This list does not thoroughly examine all possibilities. S2 lesions have similar effects as S1, and S3 and S4 lesions mainly involve the groin and genital areas, respectively.

SENSORY EXAMINATION

A sensory examination should start with a cursory scan of sensation, in which the assessor runs their hands firmly over the patient's skin bilaterally. This can be done with the patient's eyes open, while the patient indicates disparities in sensation between affected and unaffected sides. The patient then closes the eyes for detailed sensory testing, in which the examiner outlines the specific area of altered sensation and associates it with known dermatomes and peripheral nerves, keeping in mind that referred pain can confuse the picture. Other common sensory tests are superficial tactile sensation testing, using cotton or a brush, and superficial pain testing (pin prick), which uses light tapping with a sharp object. The latter tests the responses of group II afferent nerve fibers, which respond to pressure, touch, or vibration. Other group II tests include placing a tuning fork against bony protuberances (vibration) and squeezing the Achilles tendon (deep pressure). Group III fibers that are associated with temperature sensation and fast pain can be evaluated by touching the patient with hot- and cold-water-filled test tubes. There are a number of tests for proprioception (sense of position) and other sensations.

COMPONENTS

Sensation testing should be done in a dermatomal pattern, meaning all the dermatomes or skin areas innervated by the different spinal nerves should be included. The sensations to be covered and means of testing are:

- **Pain**: Evaluated by asking patient to distinguish between dull and sharp stimuli, typically a pen cap or pin.
- **Pressure**: Done by applying firm finger pressure to see if patient feels it.
- **Light touch**: Is similar to pressure except light pressure (finger, cotton ball, cloth) is applied.
- **Proprioception**: Evaluated by gripping the distal interphalangeal joints in hand or foot and asking patient to identify whether the joint is moving up or down.
- **Vibration**: Done by placing activated tuning fork on bony prominence and having patient indicate when vibration slows and stops.
- **Temperature**: Uses test tubes filled with warm or cold water placed against the body.
- **Stereognosis**: Employs a familiar object placed in patient's hand for identification.
- **Two-point discrimination**: Uses a caliper or drafting compass on the area requiring the patient to identify two points of contact within close range to one another.
- **Graphesthesia**: Done by tracing a letter or number in patient's palm for identification.
- **Double simultaneous stimulation**: Evaluated by asking patient to identify two points being touched simultaneously.

SCANNING EXAMINATION

A scanning examination is a combination of a scan of peripheral joints, myotome testing, and a sensory scan. Both upper limb and lower limb scans are done. A scanning examination is useful for differentiating between spinal-derived referred pain and pain specific to a peripheral joint. The examination involves doing a few strategic movements at each joint, including those likely to exacerbate symptoms based on history, followed by testing of key myotomes or muscles related to specific nerve roots, and then sensory scanning. Possible parts of the sensory scan are tests for reflexes, determination of the distribution of dermatomes and peripheral nerves, and neurodynamic tests. A scanning examination is a normal part of cervical and lumbar spinal assessment, but here it is also used as part of peripheral assessment. Tests specific to the peripheral joint (reflexes, sensory tests) are performed for clarification as opposed to tests for specific spinal areas if spinal involvement is suggested.

DIFFERENTIATING BETWEEN DAMAGE TO PERIPHERAL NERVES AND CONTRACTILE TISSUES

Pain, weakness, and other symptoms in an area could be due to damage to the contractile tissues or the peripheral nerves associated with them. Thus, it is important to recognize signs of peripheral nerve damage. Neurapraxia, axonotmesis, and neurotmesis are all associated with muscle weakness or muscle wasting but are neural in origin. Axonotmesis and neurotmesis can result in motor losses, such as reflex loss, joint instability, decreased range of motion, and others; sensory deficits, such as loss of vasomotor tone, depressed or abnormal sensations, skin and nail changes, and ulcerations; and sympathetic losses like dryness due to depression of sweat glands and loss of the pilomotor response. If a patient has combined sensory and motor loss, nervous tissue lesions should be suspected and the areas of loss should be examined to determine the origin.

NEURODYNAMIC TESTS

Neurodynamic, or neural tension, tests are exercises that put neural tissue under tension to potentially duplicate symptoms a patient may be experiencing. They are done to pinpoint whether a particular mechanical malfunction is due to stretching of a specific peripheral nerve or nerve root. Examples of these neurodynamic tests are the straight leg raise, the slump test, and the upper limb tension test. The basic operating principle of these tests is that neural tissue shifts toward the associated joint at the start of elongation, creating tension points. If there is nerve damage, the patient will experience tension and discomfort. The test is deemed positive if the patient's symptoms are mimicked during performance, if there is an asymmetric response, or if the patient's reaction is changed with movement of a distal body part.

NEUROLOGICAL DIAGNOSTIC TESTS
LUMBAR PUNCTURE

A lumbar puncture (LP) is a procedure in which cerebrospinal fluid (CSF) is collected using a needle inserted into the subarachnoid space at lumbar level L1 or lower in the vertebra, usually between L3 and L4. The patient lies on the side during the collection. Numerous tubes of CSF are collected to test for characteristics like color, pH, cytology, and certain substances. Results of CSF testing are used to differentiate potential causes of neurologic dysfunction, including issues such as CNS metastases from tumors, cerebral hemorrhage, meningitis, encephalitis, demyelinating disorders like multiple sclerosis, etc. LP is also used to dispense spinal anesthetic, drain CSF in patients with hydrocephalus, and instill therapeutic or diagnostic agents. Potential complications of lumbar puncture include headache, backache, high temperature, site bleeding, and trouble voiding.

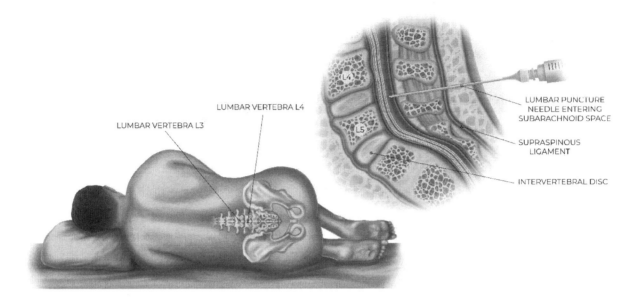

ELECTROENCEPHALOGRAPHY, EVOKED POTENTIALS, ELECTROMYOGRAPHY, AND NEVER CONDUCTION VELOCITY STUDIES

Electroencephalography (EEG), evoked potentials (EP), electromyography (EMG), and nerve conduction velocity studies all involve electrical responses in some way:

- In **EEG**, electrodes are attached to a patient's scalp to record electrical brain activity. EEG shows characteristic patterns for certain neurologic conditions, for example, seizures in epilepsy show rapid, spiking waves.
- **EPs** involve placing electrodes over parts of the brain or brain stem, applying an appropriate stimulus, and looking for conduction delays of the generated electrical responses, which can indicate lesions or tumors along that sensory pathway.
- In **EMG**, muscles are electrically stimulated and their activity documented.
- In **nerve conduction studies**, the conduction times and amplitudes of electrical response along peripheral nerves are quantified.

EMG and nerve conduction studies are generally combined to distinguish muscle diseases from peripheral nerve injury.

IMAGING TECHNIQUES

Most post-traumatic imaging done for assessment is computed tomography (CT) and/or magnetic resonance imaging (MRI). A brain or head CT is useful for identifying intracranial hemorrhage, cerebral aneurysm, etc. It is considered by many to be the definitive test for distinguishing between hemorrhagic and ischemic processes due to a cerebrovascular accident (CVA) to determine whether tissue plasminogen activator (tPA) should be administered. Other variations include CT scanning of the spine and xenon CT, in which xenon gas is inhaled and cerebral blood flow measured. Some prefer MRI for imaging, as it provides better contrast, or a variation called magnetic resonance angiography. Simple radiography may be used as well. Other techniques are cerebral angiography, in which a radiopaque contrast medium is instilled via catheter and a radiograph taken; positron emission tomography (PET), in which radioactive chemicals are injected; digital-subtraction angiography (DSA), using contrast dye, radiography, and computer subtraction; myelography; and transesophageal or transthoracic echocardiography. Ultrasound is used to look at blood flow, either low frequency in transcranial Doppler sonography or high frequency in carotid duplex ultrasound.

Neuromuscular Diseases/Conditions that Impact Effective Treatment

CLASSIFICATIONS OF NERVE INJURIES

The most frequently used classification of nerve injuries is Seddon's system which grades them into three categories:

- **Neurapraxia** is a temporary (minutes to days) physiological block initiated by pressure or stretch of the nerve. There is no axonal injury and, therefore, no wallerian degeneration. The individual experiences pain, numbness, muscle weakness, and some loss of proprioception.
- Nerve injuries that significantly damage the axons and cause wallerian degeneration but preserve the internal structure of the nerve are known as **axonotmesis**. This person experiences pain, muscle weakness, and a complete loss of motor, sensory, and sympathetic nerve functions. Sensation returns before motor functioning, and total recovery takes months.
- **Neurotmesis** occurs when the structure of the nerve is actually destroyed because it has been severed, severely scarred, or significantly compressed at length. The person with neurotmesis experiences no pain as there is anesthesia, but otherwise symptoms are similar to axonotmesis, namely muscle wasting and complete loss of motor, sensory, and sympathetic functions. Recovery requires surgery and takes months.

TRAUMATIC BRAIN INJURIES

Traumatic brain injuries (TBIs) are generally described in terms of their location, extent, and severity and the mechanism of injury:

- The location of a TBI is the cranium alone, the cranium and brain structures, or brain structures alone. TBI location is often differentiated as closed, in which protective mechanisms are maintained; open, where they are altered; **coup**, meaning the lesion is deep relative to the impact site; **contrecoup**, where the lesion and impact site are on opposite sides; or combined **coup-contrecoup**.

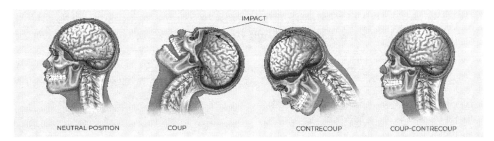

- Ways of classifying the extent include primary versus secondary (direct brain changes alone versus further complications) or focal versus diffuse, meaning specific or gross lesions.

- Severity is usually defined in terms of cognitive deficits or the Glasgow Coma Scale and diagnostic tests.
- The mechanism of injury refers to the type of force causing the damage, which is generally either acceleration-deceleration, rotational, or direct impact.

TYPES OF TBIS DUE TO SECONDARY ACCELERATION-DECELERATION FORCES

Common types of traumatic brain injuries (TBIs) due to secondary acceleration-deceleration forces are:

- **Cerebral concussion**: This is a shaking of the brain. It is characterized clinically by a transitory loss of consciousness or state of confusion, headache, faintness, irritability, inappropriate laughter, nausea, diminished concentration and memory, amnesia, and/or altered gait.
- **Cerebral contusion**: This is a slight hemorrhage to the brain. It can also occur after a skull fracture. Symptomatically, it resembles a cerebral concussion except there may be a lag period before presentation.
- **Post-concussive syndrome (PCS)**: This is a syndrome in which clinical findings are consistent with cerebral concussion, persisting for weeks or months, also including sleep disturbances and depression.
- **Cerebral laceration**: This is a tear of the cortical surface. It is usually found in association with cerebral contusion near bony surfaces. Clinical signs are variable depending on area implicated, intracranial pressure, and mass effect.
- **Diffuse axonal injury (DAI)**: This is pervasive shearing of white matter, usually after a motor vehicle accident. Its severity is defined in terms of how long the person remains in a coma, its main clinical finding. Severe DAI also presents as abnormal posturing.

HEMATOMAS FORMED POST-TBI

A hematoma is a semi-solid mass or accumulation of blood in tissues. There are three common types of hematomas that occur after a traumatic brain injury. Each is defined by the area of the brain where the blood has accumulated:

- The first is an **epidural hematoma (EDH),** in which blood accumulates in the epidural space after tearing of meningeal arteries usually due to cranial fractures.
- Another is a **subdural hematoma (SDH),** blood accretion in the subdural space due to tears in cerebral veins, intracranial hemorrhage, or excessive bleeding from a cerebral contusion. SDH can occur acutely or as late as several months after the precipitating event.
- Lastly, an **intracerebral hematoma (ICH)** is blood accumulation in the brain tissues. ICH can be caused by acceleration-deceleration forces after injury, shearing of cortical blood vessels, fractures, hypertension, or delayed bleeding.

All three of these types of hematomas present similarly, with possible clinical findings of headache, altered consciousness, contralateral hemiparesis, posture issues, etc. With EDH or SDH, the patient may have a lucid period between two bouts of loss of consciousness.

SECONDARY COMPLICATIONS

Common secondary complications from traumatic brain injuries (TBI) include increased intracranial pressure (ICP), anoxia, and seizures:

- **Increased ICP** occurs in the majority of patients with a TBI because the skull cannot adapt to the large fluid volumes resulting from edema or hemorrhage. Possible sequelae from ICP include compression of brain tissue, decreased blood flow to brain tissues, herniation, unresponsiveness, impaired consciousness, headache, high blood pressure, low heart rate, and others.
- Neurons in the hippocampus, cerebellum, and basal ganglia are susceptible to the effects of **anoxia**, or inadequate oxygenation; thus, disorders like amnesia and movement problems that are associated with these areas of the brain are common.
- **Posttraumatic epilepsy or seizures** usually occur in patients with a TBI who had open head injuries or subdural hematoma or who are older, and events are usually set off by some type of trigger, such as stress, infection, or electrolyte imbalance. Common seizure medications include phenytoin, phenobarbital, and carbamazepine.

CLINICAL PROBLEMS ASSOCIATED WITH TBIS

Traumatic brain injury patients often have a decreased level of consciousness. They also generally have various cognitive deficits, such as memory loss or disorientation. The most common motor deficits seen are abnormal postures, either decerebrate or decorticate rigidity. Other possible motor deficits include generalized weakness, tonic and primitive reflexes that cannot be controlled, balance problems, ataxia, and impaired motor sequencing. Certain senses may be impaired or lost. Communication is difficult due to abnormal tone or posturing. Many patients develop personality or psychological problems. In addition, many patients with TBI have other injuries that need to be considered.

SPINAL CORD INJURIES

A spinal cord injury (SCI) is generally described in terms of its location, mechanism of action, and, often, severity. The location is the level of the spinal cord lesion in the cervical, thoracic, or lumbar spine. Functional deficits associated with the different lesion levels are spontaneous breathing (C4), shoulder shrugging (C5), elbow flexion (C6), elbow extension (C7), finger flexion (C8 to T1), use of intercostal and abdominal muscles (T1 to T12), hip flexion (L1 to L2), hip adduction (L3), hip abduction (L4), dorsiflexion of foot (L5), plantar flexion of foot (S1 to S2), and rectal sphincter tone (S2 to S4). Possible mechanisms of injury include forward hyperflexion, hyperextension, axial compression, rotation, contusion, laceration, and transection. Forward hyperflexion and hyperextension can both cause disc herniation and vertebral dislocation or fracture, plus discontinuity in posterior or anterior spinal ligaments, respectively.

AMERICAN SPINAL INJURY IMPAIRMENT SCALE

Spinal cord injuries from trauma or impingement usually result in some level of paraplegia or quadriplegia, the inability to move the lower body or all four limbs, respectively. Spinal cord injury

(SCI) severity is usually classified according to the American Spinal Injury Association Impairment Scale in terms of motor and sensory function retained. The classifications are:

Class	Motor and Sensory Function Retained
A	Complete, no sensory or motor function in S4 to S5
B	Incomplete, maintenance of sensory function but no motor function below neurologic level, including S4 to S5
C	Incomplete, motor function preserved below neurologic level with majority of key muscles functioning at < 3/5
D	Incomplete, similar to C except most key muscles function ≥ 3/5
E	Normal, intact sensory and motor functions

SECONDARY SPINAL CORD INJURIES

Secondary spinal cord injury is the collection of pathological problems that can occur subsequent to a spinal cord injury (SCI). Much of secondary SCI is vascular in nature, including possible vasospasm in spinal blood vessels, intraparenchymal hemorrhage, and breakdown of the barrier between blood and the brain and spinal cord. The patient goes into neurogenic shock and loses the ability to autoregulate functions. Other complications include increasing calcium levels, which stimulate free radicals, leading to further tissue damage. The neurologic substances catecholamines and opioids are discharged, and microglia and macrophages accumulate. Immediately after a SCI, the injured person experiences spinal shock, hypotension, bradycardia, and hypothermia. Later, physiological sequelae can include autonomic dysreflexia, orthostatic hypotension, impaired functions (respiratory, bladder, bowel, sexual), deep venous thrombosis, diabetes insipidus, SIADH, etc.

INCOMPLETE SPINAL CORD INJURY SYNDROMES

Incomplete spinal cord injury syndromes include:

- **Central cord syndrome**: Impingement of the central cord through a hyperextension injury, presence of a tumor, rheumatoid arthritis, or a cyst within the spinal cord (syringomyelia); lesion applies pressure to anterior horn cells, causing bilateral motor paralysis primarily in the upper extremities, sensory losses, and sometimes bowel and bladder dysfunction.
- **Anterior cord syndrome**: Damage to anterior cord via a hyperflexion injury, disc herniation, or damage to an anterior spinal artery; causes damage to the anterolateral spinothalamic and cortical spinal tracts and the anterior horn, resulting in bilateral loss of pain and temperature sensations and most motor functions.
- **Brown-Sequard syndrome**: Damage to half of the spinal cord due to things like stab wounds, epidural hematoma, cervical spondylosis, etc.; patient loses sensations of pain and temperature on the opposite side, and on the same side, losses include sensations of touch, proprioception, and vibration and motor function.
- **Dorsal column or posterior cord syndrome**: Compression of posterior spinal artery from tumor or infarct; bilateral deficits in senses of vibration and proprioception.
- **Cauda equina injuries**: Due to fracture or dislocation below L1; may cause flaccidity, areflexia, loss of excretory functions.

MANAGEMENT

Medically, a patient with a spinal cord injury (SCI) is stabilized, including ventilatory support and treatment for secondary injuries as needed. The patient is immobilized, using a collar, orthosis, traction, halo vest, and/or surgical fusion of fragments, and generally given methylprednisolone promptly to enhance blood flow and decrease possible tissue damage. For symptoms of autonomic dysreflexia (in injuries above T6), such as significant hypertension, pounding headache, etc., patients are given medications to lower blood pressure (nitroglycerin patch, vasodilators, nifedipine). Patients with postural hypotension are managed with fluids, abdominal binders, or appropriate drugs. Associated pain is usually dysesthetic (phantom) pain, addressed with NSAIDS, antiepileptics, anticonvulsants, tricyclic antidepressants, or psychological techniques. Pressure ulcers are addressed with pressure-relief techniques. Heterotopic ossification of nearby bones is managed with etidronate, range-of-motion exercises, and, sometimes, surgical resection. If contractures develop, a good stretching program is indicated. Patients may be given oral warfarin or IV heparin to prevent deep vein thrombosis.

ADDRESSING RESPIRATORY COMPROMISE

Patients with high cervical spinal cord injuries often cannot breathe independently because they are paralyzed or their diaphragm, usually innervated by nerve roots C3 to C5, is weak. Lower-level injuries can also cause respiratory compromise as other breathing-related muscles may be affected, such as the external intercostals innervated starting at the T1 level, upper abdominals at T7 to T9, and lower abdominals at T9 to T11. Injuries below T12 should not affect respiration. If there is respiratory compromise, possible interventions include use of abdominal binders, upright positioning, assisted cough techniques, diaphragmatic strengthening exercises, and incentive spirometry.

ADDRESSING BLADDER, BOWEL, AND SEXUAL DYSFUNCTION

The bladder is innervated by spinal nerves at the S2 to S4 sacral. It is flaccid or areflexic during the initial spinal shock after injury and remains so in patients whose injury is to the cauda equina or conus medullaris, the terminal end of the spinal cord. These patients have a flaccid or non-reflexive bladder, which necessitates manual emptying. However, if the injury is above the S2 level, the patient will have a reflex or spastic bladder, which they can induce to empty through external stimulation. Bladder training is a key component of therapy. The anal sphincter is innervated at the S2 level, and patients may have bowel problems as well. Correspondingly, a regular bowel program, high-fiber diet, fluids, stool softeners, and/or manual stimulation are generally indicated. In terms of sexual dysfunction, the main problem for males is limitation of the ability to ejaculate, which makes them less fertile. Women can become pregnant but cannot feel uterine contractions during labor. The therapist's role is basically informational in this case.

ADDRESSING SPASTICITY

Spasticity, or muscle hypertonicity, is a common complication in spinal cord injuries. It is probably due to lingering effects of supraspinal centers and inadequate modulation of spinal pathways. The presence of spasticity is both good and bad because while it is annoying to the patient and others, it also facilitates muscle bulking, prevents muscle atrophy, and helps circulation. Appropriate physical therapy interventions for spasticity include weight bearing, static stretching, correct positioning, cryotherapy, electrical stimulation, and aquatic exercises. A common drug given for spasticity is baclofen, administered orally or via an intrathecal pump. Other pharmacologic agents include botulinum toxin A injections into the muscle (causing its temporary paralysis); injectable phenol as a nerve block; and oral diazepam, tizanidine, or dantrolene sodium. Spasticity can also be addressed surgically. Surgical procedures include neurectomy, excision of a portion of the nerve; rhizotomy, resection of a dorsal or sensory nerve; myelotomy, cutting of spinal cord tracts; and tenotomy, tendon release.

CEREBROVASCULAR ACCIDENTS

A cerebrovascular accident (CVA), or stroke, is the sudden onset of neurologic signs resulting from blockage or rupture of a blood vessel in the brain. It is often preceded days or months in advance by a transient ischemic attack (TIA), a focal brain or retinal disturbance of short duration.

The majority of strokes are **ischemic CVAs**, meaning there is decreased oxygenation to the brain due to a poor blood supply. This type of CVA is further characterized as either thrombotic, due to blood vessel constriction (for example, atherosclerosis), or embolic, due to a clot lodged in a cerebral blood vessel. Cerebral tissue in the area undergoes infarct or death, adjacent neurons are injured, and other substances are released that cause additional cellular damage.

The other common type of CVA is a **hemorrhagic CVA,** in which there is excessive bleeding due to rupture of a cerebral blood vessel, again causing cerebral hypoperfusion. Hemorrhagic CVAs are most commonly caused by factors such as hypertension and vessel malformations, in addition to trauma. A rarer type observed is a lacunar CVA, which is an infarction in a small vessel in regions like the basal ganglia and thalamus; this type is seen primarily in patients with diabetes and hypertension and does not cause cognitive or visual deficits.

NEUROLOGIC SIGNS OF CVA'S BASED ON THE ARTERIES AFFECTED

Arteries in the brain affected by a cerebrovascular accident and the corresponding neurologic signs are as follows:

- **Internal carotid artery**: Blindness on one side; hemiplegia and hemianesthesia on the opposing side; significant aphasia (inability to produce and understand speech)
- **Middle cerebral artery**: Altered speech, cognition, mobility, and sensation; contralateral hemiplegia or hemiparesis; motor and sensory loss; and visual field losses
- **Anterior cerebral artery**: Amnesia, personality changes, confusion; bladder incontinence; contralateral hemiplegic or hemiparesis
- **Posterior cerebral artery**: Hemianesthesia; ataxia; tremors; memory loss; aphasia; vision problems; hemiplegia on opposite side
- **Posterior inferior cerebellar artery**: Difficulty swallowing and speaking; anesthesia for pain and temperature in face and cornea on ipsilateral side and trunk and extremities on contralateral side
- **Anterior inferior and superior cerebellar arteries**: Articulation and gross movement problems; nystagmus
- **Vertebral or basilar arteries**: Signs are dependent on amount of occlusion, ranging from weakness and other sensory and motor deficits to coma; if in anterior portion of the pons, "Locked-in" Syndrome occurs, characterized by complete lack of movement, except for eyelids

DIAGNOSIS AND ACUTE MANAGEMENT

The patient experiencing a cerebrovascular accident (CVA) should be hospitalized. The physician performs a physical examination that includes neurological tests for motor and sensory functions, reflexes, and speech. Imaging is done to determine whether the brain vessel damage causing CVA is ischemic or hemorrhagic. Common imaging techniques used are magnetic resonance imaging or computed tomography. Acute medical management is directed at regulating the person's blood pressure, cerebral perfusion, and intracranial pressure. Patients are usually given the anticoagulant heparin, diuretics, calcium channel blockers, prophylactic anticonvulsants, and the antithrombolytic tissue plasminogen activator (tPA), if the stroke is ischemic. Patients with hemorrhagic CVAs often require surgical procedures, such as evacuation of the hematoma, removal of a blood vessel, or placement of a metal clip at the base of an aneurysm. Unproven treatment options include administration of cytoprotective drugs like calcium channel blockers, injection of fibrinolytic agents via a catheter, use of mechanical clot removal devices, and application of mild to moderate hypothermia to preserve neurologic function.

BRUNNSTROM STAGES OF RECOVERY FOLLOWING A CVA

Brunnstrom identified seven stages of motor recovery by patients who have had a cerebrovascular accident:

Stage	Function
I	Flaccidity, in which the patient has no voluntary or reflex activity in the involved extremity.
II	The period when spasticity and synergy patterns begin to develop. In Brunnstrom's view, synergy patterns involve characteristic groups of muscles that work together to create movement patterns, for example, flexion versus extension of the same region.
III	The period where spasticity increases and peaks, during which movement synergies of the involved extremity can be executed voluntarily.
IV	The patient can deviate from characteristic synergy patterns and perform some combined movements.
V	Synergy patterns are less evident and the patient can perform more complex combined movements.
VI	Spasticity has vanished and the individual can perform isolated and combined movements.
VII	Characterized by a return to normal function and renewed ability to perform fine motor skills.

COMMON IMPAIRMENTS POST-CVA

After a stroke, patients usually have flaccid muscles, followed by a period of spasticity, before recovery of motor skills. Spasticity is often developed at first in the shoulder and pelvic girdles, resulting in characteristic posturing. Patients have difficulty with processes requiring strength, such as gripping, and may exhibit apraxia, the inability to perform complex movements. They have sensory, communication, and/or orofacial impairments. Aphasia occurs in about 30% of patients who've experienced stroke in the form of Broca's aphasia, where they have trouble with expression; Wernicke's aphasia, where they cannot understand what is being said; or global aphasia, which encompasses both. Orofacial deficits include facial asymmetries, dysphagia (difficulty swallowing), and inability to coordinate eating and breathing. Patients usually have respiratory problems, in particular decreased lung expansion and volumes due to lessened ability to control respiratory muscles. Primitive spinal and brain stem reflexes are recalled, and patients may have associated reactions. Deep tendon reflexes may be absent or exaggerated, depending on whether they are in a flaccid or spastic phase. Common initial problems are bowel and bladder dysfunction.

PRIMITIVE SPINAL AND BRAIN STEM REFLEXES POST-CVA

Patients revert to the use of primitive, non-voluntary spinal and brain stem reflexes when their central nervous system is damaged. Common spinal level reflexes are:

- **Flexor withdrawal**: Extension of the toes with ankle dorsiflexion when a stimulus is applied to the bottom of the foot.
- **Cross-extension**: Flexion followed by extension of opposing extremity after application of stimulus to ball of foot when leg is extended.

- **Startle**: Extension and abduction of the upper extremities in response to an unexpected loud noise.
- **Grasp**: Flexion of the toes or fingers when pressure is applied to the ball of the foot or palm of the hand, respectively.

Primitive brain stem reflexes include:

- **Symmetric tonic neck reflex**: Where flexion or extension of the neck results in similar response in arms but opposite in legs.
- **Asymmetric tonic neck reflex**: Where rotation of the neck to one side results in extension of the same side arm and leg, and flexion of the arm and leg on the opposite side.
- **Tonic labyrinthine reflex**: In which lying prone or supine encourages flexion or extension, respectively.
- **Tonic thumb reflex**: In which elevation of the involved extremity causes thumb extension with the forearm in supination.

Associated reactions are automatic movements in other parts of the body in response to active or resisted movements.

COMPLICATIONS POST-CVA

Development of contractures and deformities is one of the most common complications of cerebrovascular accident, due primarily to the spasticity present after a stroke. The vast majority of patients with hemiplegia develop shoulder pain and, often, loss of function caused by either muscle weakness or spasticity. Complex regional pain syndrome (CRPS) often occurs. CRPS is a three-stage process developing over the course of six months to a year, in which initially the person has burning and aching pain, edema, warm skin, and fast hair and nail growth; which develops into joint stiffness, brittle nails, and cool skin; and eventually, into irreparable skin changes and contractures. Patients who have had CVA are also prone to falls, thrombophlebitis, joint and muscle pain, and depression.

CEREBRAL ANEURYSM, AV MALFORMATION, AND SUBARACHNOID HEMORRHAGE

A cerebral aneurysm is a localized ballooning or dilation of a cerebral blood vessel due to weakness in its wall. Causes include congenital defects, high blood pressure, atherosclerosis, and trauma. An arteriovenous malformation (AVM) is an abnormal connection between arteries and veins without capillary interface. AVM is usually congenital and can cause signs like headache, paralysis, epilepsy, and sensory deficits. Both cerebral aneurysms and AVMs can lead to bleeding complications in the brain, making them primary mechanisms (along with tumors, trauma, and infections) for subarachnoid hemorrhage (SAH), one type of hemorrhagic cerebrovascular accident in which blood accumulates in the subarachnoid space. Low-grade SAH may be asymptomatic or present simply as headache and neck rigidity, but increasing severity is characterized by further neurological deficits and the possibility of coma. Management of SAH may include surgical intervention, such as aneurysm repair with blood evacuation, and various measures to stabilize the patient. Common complications are further bleeding, hydrocephalus, seizure, and vasospasm, which can lead to tissue damage and sensory alterations.

DEMENTIA

Dementia is a chronic condition in which there is progressive and irreversible loss of memory and function. There are many types of dementia that may be encountered:

1. **Creutzfeldt-Jakob disease**: Rapidly progressive dementia with impaired memory, behavioral changes, and incoordination
2. **Dementia with Lewy Bodies**: Similar to Alzheimer's, but symptoms may fluctuate frequently; may also include visual hallucinations, muscle rigidity, and tremors
3. **Frontotemporal dementia**: Causes marked changes in personality and behavior; characterized by difficulty using and understanding language
4. **Mixed dementia**: Combination of different types of dementia
5. **Normal pressure hydrocephalus**: Characterized by ataxia, memory loss, and urinary incontinence
6. **Parkinson's dementia**: Involves impaired decision making and difficulty concentrating, learning new material, understanding complex language, and sequencing
7. **Vascular dementia**: Memory loss less pronounced than that common to Alzheimer's, but symptoms are similar

Physical therapy considerations include reduction of distractions, simplification of instructions, and completion of transfers in a manner that will reduce the patient's fear of falling.

HYDROCEPHALUS

Hydrocephalus is the abnormal accumulation of cerebrospinal fluid (CSF) in the ventricles or cavities of the brain. This usually causes increased intracranial pressure, head enlargement, headache, convulsions, and/or altered consciousness. There are two types. The first is noncommunicating, or obstructive, hydrocephalus, which is caused by an obstruction to CSF flow in the ventricular system. The other is communicating hydrocephalus, in which the obstruction is at the border of the subarachnoid space. Hydrocephalus is managed by addressing the underlying cause, if possible, or using shunts to divert the accumulating CSF. Some communicating hydrocephalus is a subset called normal-pressure hydrocephalus (NHP), in which there is no increase in intracranial pressure. NHP is characterized by confusion, gait changes, and urinary incontinence; it is usually improved with a lumbar puncture to remove surplus CSF or placement of a ventriculoperitoneal shunt.

SEIZURES

A seizure is an abrupt-onset of aberrant neurologic functioning due to excessive neuronal activation in the cerebral cortex or deep limbic. Epilepsy is a recurrent form. Underlying causes of seizure include cerebrovascular accidents, head trauma or surgery, and meningitis. Seizures are classified as partial, if they occur focally in one hemisphere, or generalized, if they derive from both hemispheres or at deep midline. Partial seizures are further divided into simple partial (no loss of consciousness), complex partial (transitory loss with motionless staring), and partial with secondary generalization (moving toward both hemispheres). Generalized seizures are categorized as tonic (abrupt flexor or extensor rigidity), clonic (rhythmic, jerky muscle movements), tonic-clonic (sudden extensor rigidity, then flexor jerking), atonic (no muscle tone), absence (transitory unresponsiveness and blank staring), and myoclonic (rapid, nonrhythmic jerking). Possible signs of seizure include aura, tremors, visual changes, hallucinations, and faintness. The definitive diagnostic tool is EEG. Management includes addressing the cause, prescribing antiepileptic drugs, resectioning the focal point, and/or embedding a vagal nerve stimulator. Status epilepticus, where seizures continue, is an emergency necessitating life support due to threats to the integrity of the individual's airway.

SYNCOPE

Syncope is the brief loss of consciousness and postural tone due to cerebral underperfusion. It is usually accompanied by slow heart rate and hypotension. Syncope has four types of origins: cardiogenic, due to drug toxicity or various types of cardiac abnormalities; neurologic, with causes like seizure, vertigo, and cerebral atherosclerosis; reflexive, due to carotid sinus syndrome or some type of vasovagal response; and orthostatic, caused by things like protracted bed rest or drug side effects. Syncope is confirmed through history, event recorders, tilt-table testing, and CT or MRI, if there is new neurologic evidence. Its management is highly dependent on the underlying cause.

POLIOMYELITIS AND POSTPOLIOMYELITIS SYNDROME

Poliomyelitis is a neuroinfectious disease, meaning it is of infectious origin, in this case caused by polioviruses spread via the fecal-oral route or through drinking contaminated water. Poliomyelitis is preventable with administration of inactivated poliovirus vaccine (IVP). There is a wide range of clinical presentation for poliomyelitis. Milder cases can be asymptomatic, a general illness without fever, or aseptic meningitis. However, more severe poliomyelitis usually presents as asymmetric paralysis of respiratory, throat, and leg muscles, along with fever and muscle pain. This paralysis may go away, have lingering effects, or lead to death. Polio is managed with administration of analgesics and fever reducers, bronchopulmonary hygiene, bed rest, and techniques to prevent contractures, such as positioning and range of motion.

Postpoliomyelitis syndrome (PPS) is a condition that occurs decades after paralytic poliomyelitis. It is due to overuse or aging of originally involved motor units and is characterized by fatigue, pain, cold intolerance, and, sometimes, muscle atrophy or inflammation. Short bouts of exercise interspersed with rest periods are suggested; aquatic exercise is a good option as it decreases stress on joints, bones, and muscles.

MENINGITIS AND ENCEPHALITIS

Meningitis and encephalitis are two neuroinfectious diseases in which there is inflammation of the meninges or brain tissues. respectively. Meningitis is spread through inhalation of infected airborne mucous droplets. Bacterial meningitis can be caused by meningococci, pneumococci, or *Haemophilus* and affects many parts of the brain, leading to high intracranial pressure, hydrocephalus, headache, neck rigidity, and, potentially, a number of other primarily neurologic complications. There is also a milder viral form. Meningitis is addressed with antibiotics, anti-infective agents, immunologic agents, analgesics, IV fluids and vasopressors to maintain blood pressure, measures to regulate intracranial pressure, and use of ventilators, if indicated.

Infectious encephalitis is mainly transmitted by herpes simplex type I virus-containing respiratory droplets. Other modes of encephalitis transmission are through bites from mosquitoes infected with another virus and nasal intake during swimming of an ameba. Symptoms of encephalitis include fever, altered consciousness and other neurologic abnormalities, severe frontal lobe headaches, hyperthermia, weakness, etc. It is treated with anti-infectives, IV fluids and electrolytes, management of intracranial pressure, mechanical ventilation, and nasogastric feeding.

VESTIBULAR DISORDERS

The vestibular system is made up of various canals and organs in the inner ear, as well as parts of the brain and spinal cord. Normally, it stabilizes visual images on the retina during movement, preserves postural stability during head movements, and maintains spatial orientation. If the system is disrupted, the patient may experience vertigo, or the sensation that the surroundings are moving or spinning. Widespread conditions associated with vestibular dysfunction include:

- **Benign positional paroxysmal vertigo (BPPV)**: Brief, severe vertigo occurring with head position changes; due primarily to some type of trauma. The Hallpike-Dix test often used to pinpoint the affected canal by observing for nystagmus and vertigo with head in different positions. Later, the Epley maneuver is used to right the patient, who should sleep that night in a semi-recumbent position
- **Acute vestibular neuronitis**: Sudden-onset, longer-lasting vertigo that is usually due to viral infection. Treatment is mainly supportive
- **Meniere's disease**: Episodes of vertigo due to end lymphatic fluid in the inner ear. Management includes salt restriction, diuretics, vestibular reducing medications, endolymphatic shunt, etc.
- **Bilateral vestibular hypofunction (BVH)**: Generally, permanent oscillating vision and unsteady gait caused by aminoglycoside drugs.

MEASURING VESTIBULAR DYSFUNCTION

The majority of the tests to measure vestibular dysfunction include some type of vision test. One is the dynamic visual acuity test (DVA), in which the patient reads the low line on the eye chart while the professional oscillates the patient's head to look for declining visual acuity. Several vision tests look for presence of nystagmus, or involuntary eyeball movement, including static ocular observation and head shaking, followed by clinician observation. Other vision tests include examination saccades, the head thrust test, the rotary chair test, caloric testing, and the Hallpike-Dix test. Absent or slowed nystagmus is indicative of pathology in many of these tests. Another somewhat different assessment tool is the Romberg test, in which the patient stands with feet together, first with eyes open and then closed, and increased sway or balance loss with the latter is suggestive of vestibular dysfunction. The sensory organization test is a six-part assessment, during which the patient stands either on a fixed or moving platform with eyes open, closed, or in front of a moving screen and sway is noted for each condition.

AMYOTROPHIC LATERAL SCLEROSIS (ALS)

Amyotrophic lateral sclerosis (ALS) is a progressive degenerative disease of the upper and lower motor neurons, resulting in progressively severe symptoms such as spasticity, hyperreflexia, muscle weakness, and paralysis that can cause dysphagia, cramping, muscular atrophy, and respiratory dysfunction. ALS may be sporadic or familial (rare). Speech may become monotone; however, cognitive functioning usually remains intact. Eventually, patients become immobile and cannot breathe independently.

Diagnosis is based on history, electromyography, nerve conduction studies, and MRI. Treatment includes riluzole to delay progression of the disease. Patients in the ED usually have been diagnosed and have developed an acute complication, such as acute respiratory failure, aspiration pneumonia, or other trauma.

Management includes:

- Nebulizer treatments with bronchodilators and steroids
- Antibiotics for infection
- Mechanical ventilation

If **ventilatory assistance** is needed, it is important to determine if the patient has a living will expressing the wish to be ventilated or not or has assigned power of attorney for health matters to someone to make this decision.

The role of physical therapy with ALS patients is to find ways for the patient to cope as well as possible with the disability, including use of adaptive equipment.

Guillain-Barre Syndrome (GBS)

Guillain-Barré syndrome (GBS) is an autoimmune disorder of the myelinated motor peripheral nervous system, causing ascending and descending paralysis. GBS is often triggered by a viral infection, but may be idiopathic in origin. Diagnosis is by history, clinical symptoms, and lumbar puncture, which often show increased protein with normal glucose and cell count although protein may not increase for a week or more.

> **Review Video: Guillain-Barre Syndrome**
> Visit mometrix.com/academy and enter code: 742900

Symptoms include:

- Numbness and tingling with increasing weakness of lower extremities that may become generalized, sometimes resulting in complete paralysis and inability to breathe without ventilatory support.
- Deep tendon reflexes are typically absent and some people experience facial weakness and ophthalmoplegia (paralysis of muscles controlling movement of eyes).

Management includes:

- Supportive: Fluids, physical therapy, and antibiotics for infections
- Patients should be hospitalized for observation and placed on ventilator support if forced vital capacity is reduced.
- While there is no definitive treatment, plasma exchange or IV immunoglobulin may shorten the duration of symptoms.
- Acute phase physical therapy includes things like postural drainage, passive range of motion, and massage. As respiratory and autonomic functions improve, acclimation to upright posture should be started, and as they recover muscle strength, short episodes of non-fatiguing exercise should be initiated.

Multiple Sclerosis

Multiple sclerosis is an autoimmune disorder of the CNS in which the myelin sheath around the nerves is damaged and replaced by scar tissue that prevents conduction of nerve impulses.

Symptoms vary widely and can include problems with balance and coordination, tremors, slurring of speech, cognitive impairment, vision impairment, nystagmus, pain, and bladder and bowel dysfunction. Symptoms may be relapsing-remitting, progressive, or a combination. Onset is usually at 20-30 years of age, with incidence higher in females. Patient may initially present with problems walking or falling or optic neuritis (30%) causing loss of central vision. Males may complain of sexual dysfunction as an early symptom. Others have dysuria with urinary retention.

Diagnosis is based on clinical and neurological examination and MRI. **Treatment** is symptomatic and includes treatment to shorten duration of episodes and slow progress.

- **Glucocorticoids**: Methylprednisolone
- **Immunomodulator**: Interferon beta, glatiramer acetate, natalizumab
- **Immunosuppressant**: Mitoxantrone
- **Hormone**: Estriol (for females)

> **Review Video: Multiple Sclerosis**
> Visit mometrix.com/academy and enter code: 417355

PARKINSON'S DISEASE

Parkinson's disease (PD) is an extrapyramidal movement motor system disorder caused by loss of brain cells that produce dopamine. Typical symptoms include tremor of face and extremities, rigidity, bradykinesia, akinesia, poor posture, and a lack of balance and coordination causing increasing problems with mobility, talking, and swallowing. Some may suffer depression and mood changes. Tremors usually present unilaterally in an upper extremity.

Diagnosis includes:

- Cogwheel rigidity test: The extremity is put through passive range of motion, which causes increased muscle tone and ratchet-like movements.
- Physical and neurological exam
- Complete history to rule out drug-induced Parkinson akinesia

Management includes:

- Symptomatic support
- Dopaminergic therapy: Levodopa, amantadine, and carbidopa
- Anticholinergics: Trihexyphenidyl, benztropine
- For drug-induced Parkinson's, terminate drugs

Drug therapy tends to decrease in effectiveness over time, and patients may present with a marked increase in symptoms. Discontinuing the drugs for 1 week may exacerbate symptoms initially, but functioning may improve when drugs are reintroduced.

CEREBRAL PALSY

Cerebral palsy (CP) is a non-progressive motor dysfunction related to CNS damage associated with congenital, hypoxic, or traumatic injury before, during, or ≤2 years after birth. It may include visual defects, speech impairment, seizures, and mental retardation. There are four **types of motor dysfunction**:

- **Spastic**: Damage to the cerebral cortex or pyramidal tract. Constant hypertonia and rigidity lead to contractures and curvature of the spine.
- **Dyskinetic**: Damage to the extrapyramidal, basal ganglia. Tremors and twisting with exaggerated posturing and impairment of voluntary muscle control.
- **Ataxic**: Damage to the extrapyramidal cerebellum. Atonic muscles in infancy with lack of balance, instability of muscles, and poor gait.
- **Mixed**: Combinations of all three types with multiple areas of damage.

Characteristics of CP include:

- Hypotonia or hypertonia with rigidity and spasticity
- Athetosis (constant writhing motions)
- Ataxia
- Hemiplegia (one-sided involvement, more severe in upper extremities)
- Diplegia (all extremities involved, but more severe in lower extremities)
- Quadriplegia (all extremities involved with arms flexed and legs extended)

MYELOMENINGOCELE

Myelomeningocele (MMC) is a congenital disorder primarily involving the nervous system in which there is defective development of the spinal cord during gestation. The defect for MMC, also known as spina bifida cystica, is an incomplete vertebral closure with a cyst containing a malformed spinal cord. The MMC is generally removed and closed surgically within the first day of birth. The main defects neurologically are motor paralysis and sensory loss below the level of the MMC. The children tend to develop certain lower-extremity deformities, particularly foot deformities, such as clubfoot. They are also prone to osteoporosis, neuropathic fractures, spinal deformities, and hydrocephalus. The hydrocephalus, or increased levels of spinal fluid in the brain, is usually but not always found in association with a prevalent associated malformation in the cerebellum, medulla, and cervical portion of the spinal cord, called Arnold-Chiari type II malformation. Thus, most MMC patients with MMC have some sort of shunt to drain the cerebrospinal fluid. They may have central nervous system deterioration, hydromyelia (excess CSF in the spinal cord) or a tethered spinal cord leading to scoliosis, various sensory impairments, bowel and bladder problems, and, interestingly, latex allergies.

GENETIC NEUROLOGIC DISORDERS IN CHILDREN

Some important genetic disorders involving the neurologic system include the following:

- **Down Syndrome**: Presence of extra 21st chromosome in bodily cells, resulting in intellectual disability, developmental delays, musculoskeletal deficits (such as instability at the atlanto-axial joint involving the two upper cervical vertebra), hypotonicity, flat facial features, a variety of neurological deficits, etc.
- **Arthropyosis multiplex congenital**: A nonprogressive neuromuscular syndrome inherited on chromosome 9 (or 5 in neurogenic form); characterized by multiple contractures.
- **Osteogenesis imperfecta**: Autonomic dominant disorder affecting collagen synthesis and bone metabolism, making individual prone to bone fractures.
- **Spinal muscle atrophy (SMA)**: Autonomic recessive, progressive neurologic disorder destroying anterior horn cells and lower motor neurons:
  - *Type I acute infantile SMA* occurs shortly after birth and is characterized by respiratory and other oral issues and a frog-leg posture.
  - *Type II chronic SMA* starts at approximately 2-18 months of age characterized by muscle weakness and scoliosis. Later-onset Kugelberg-Welander SMA is similar.
- **Duchenne muscular dystrophy (DMD)**: X-linked recessive trait in which muscle protein dystrophin is absent; symptomatic only in boys, presenting as progressive weakness (including cardiac and respiratory muscles), diminished range of motion, and contractures.
- **Fragile X syndrome**: Presence of fragile site on X chromosome; signified by intellectual disability and other neurologic defects.

Physical Therapy Interventions

FRENKEL EXERCISES

Frenkel exercises are a set of movements done in supine, sitting, or standing position. They are designed to be done slowly and evenly to improve coordination. Typically, there are eight supine movements in the set, involving different combinations of lower-extremity flexions, extensions, abductions, adductions, and/or heel sliding. There are four sitting-position Frenkel exercises, which address issues like sitting steadily, rising, and sitting down, etc. There are four more exercises done standing, three of which involve walking along a winding strip, between two parallel lines, or along a floor tracing. Frenkel exercises are good interventions for patients with ataxia, such as those with multiple sclerosis.

PROPRIOCEPTIVE NEUROMUSCULAR FACILITATION

Proprioceptive neuromuscular facilitation (PNF) is a physical therapy intervention strategy that focuses on improving functional performance through increasing strength, flexibility, and range of motion. The goals of PNF are to help the patient develop head and trunk control, begin and sustain movement, manage shifts in center of gravity, and control the trunk and pelvis at midline while moving extremities. PNF expounds that there are 10 components to this improved motor learning:

- **Manual contacts**: Application of hands to the skin over the target muscle groups in the direction of preferred movement.
- **Mirroring**: Therapist mimicking of the patient's body position and mechanics.
- **Use of stretch**: Facilitation of muscle activity.
- **Manual resistance**: Minimization of internal resistance and application of external resistance.
- **Irradiation**: The concept that muscle activity spreads out or overflows from the point of resistance.
- **Facilitation of joints through traction and approximation.**
- **Timing or sequencing** of movement.
- **Use of diagonal patterns** of movement.
- Use of **visual cues**.
- **Concise verbal input in three phases**: Preparation, action, and correction.

UPPER-EXTREMITY PATTERNS

One basic tenet of PNF is the use of diagonal combinations of joint movements, called patterns. The therapist aids the patient through manual contact and other principles of PNF. Extremity patterns are designated in terms of the direction of movement at the proximal joint, the resultant movement, and directions for flexion and extension. Upper-extremity (UE) patterns are either diagonal 1 (D1) or 2 (D2), depending on whether the pattern moves counterclockwise or clockwise, respectively. The flexion or extension designation describes the starting position for the joint in question. The pattern starts in flexion or extension, goes through some sequence of internal or external rotation, plus adduction or abduction. Below are examples of the four upper extremity patters for the shoulder:

- **UE-D1 Flexion pattern** is shoulder flexion/adduction/external rotation.
- **UE-D1 Extension pattern** is shoulder extension/abduction/internal rotation.
- **UE-D2 Flexion pattern** is shoulder flexion/abduction/external rotation.
- **UE-D2 Extension pattern** is shoulder extension/adduction/internal rotation.

Flexion patterns always involve shoulder external rotation, forearm supination, and radial wrist deviation, while extension patterns involve shoulder internal rotation, forearm pronation, and ulnar wrist deviation. UE patterns are combined in the lifting and reverse lifting and chopping patterns.

LOWER-EXTREMITY PATTERNS

Lower-extremity (LE) patterns for PNF are named similarly to upper-extremity patterns, for example, LE-D1 flexion and so on, with D1 patterns moving counterclockwise and D2 ones moving clockwise. Here, hip internal rotation is always paired with abduction and hip external rotation with adduction. In addition, the patient also goes through a posterior or anterior pelvic tilt during the pattern. The main patterns for the hip are:

- **LE-D1 Flexion**: Hip flexion/adduction/external rotation, basically plantar flexion of the foot and pulling the leg across.
- **LE-D1 Extension**: Hip extension/abduction/internal rotation.
- **LE-D2 Flexion**: Hip flexion/abduction/internal rotation.
- **LE-D2 Extension**: Hip extension/adduction/external rotation.

SCAPULAR AND PELVIC PATTERNS

Scapular patterns are somewhat unique because they take into account scapulohumeral biomechanics. They begin in elevation or depression and end in the opposite. Elevation, a type of flexion, is when the scapula, or shoulder, is pulled up or shrugged, and depression is a type of extension in which it is depressed and retracted downward. Both can be done to the anterior or posterior side with the patient side-lying.

Pelvic patterns are analogous in that there is a limited range of motion in the pelvis, the patterns are similarly named, and side-lying positions (with flexed legs) are generally used. Here, the most germane patterns are the anterior elevation and posterior depression pelvic patterns, which involve pulling the pelvis up and forward or back into the therapist's, respectively.

TECHNIQUES THAT ADDRESS MOBILITY AND STABILITY

PNF techniques that address mobility and stability include the following:

- **Rhythmic initiation**: Focuses on enhancing mobility by sequentially introducing passive, active-assisted, and, eventually, active or slightly resisted movements.
- **Rhythmic rotation**: Applies passive movements in a rotational fashion to encourage relaxation, reduce tone and lessen spasticity, and, ultimately, improve joint mobility.
- **Hold-relax active movement**: Consists of sequences of resisted isometric contraction, followed by relaxation and incremental lengthening of position; goal is to increase range of motion.
- **Hold-relax**: Essentially the same as hold-relax active movement, except usually includes verbal cues; patient-controlled movement is ideal.
- **Contract relax**: Uses resisted isotonic or isometric contraction of a short muscle to available range of motion (ROM), followed by verbal instruction to move it further, hold for a least five seconds, and then relax; used to increase ROM.
- **Alternating isometrics**: Therapist uses manual contact or resistance alternately, against opposing muscle groups, to enhance stability, strength, and endurance in them; also involves verbal cues to maintain stability.
- **Rhythmic stabilization**: Primarily promotes stability by simultaneous contraction of muscles around the target joint, while applying a rotary force.

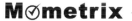

TECHNIQUES THAT ADDRESS CONTROLLED MOBILITY OR SKILL DEVELOPMENT

PNF techniques that address controlled mobility or skill development include:

- **Slow reversal**: Uses concentric contraction of muscles and reversal of manual contacts at the end of range of motion to the other direction to develop smooth transitions.
- **Slow reversal hold**: Variation of slow reversal, in which a resisted isometric contraction is held before reversing direction; useful for moving from emphasis on stability to mobility, as well as controlled mobility and skill.
- **Agonistic reversals**: Involves concentric contraction of muscle, an isometric hold against resistance, eccentric contraction through resistance during return to baseline position, and holding at the end; primarily promotes functional stability in a controlled manner; bridging exercise is a good example.
- **Resisted progression**: Application of resistance during perfection of a skill, such as creeping or walking.

PHYSICAL THERAPY INTERVENTIONS FOR CVA'S

EARLY PHYSICAL THERAPY INTERVENTIONS

An important consideration with patients post-CVA is positioning, which should rotate between supine, with support on the involved side under the patient's scapula, pelvis, and knee; side-lying on the uninvolved side, with involved leg and arm crossed over and supported by pillows; and side-lying on the involved side, with involved affected shoulder forward and protracted, forearm in supination, and, again, support. The patient should be assisted with bridging, pushing the hips upward, and bridging with approximation or compression applied through the knee. Early types of bedside interventions include hip extension over the edge of the bed or other surface, straight leg raises with the uninvolved extremity, lower trunk rotation in hook lying position, hip and knee flexion while supine, separation and pushing against the patient's toes to inhibit toe clawing and promote ankle dorsiflexion, scapular mobilization (all of which involve manual contact by the physical therapist or assistant), and double arm elevation by the patient alone. Use of facilitation techniques is, for the most part, controversial or unproven. Inhibition techniques, such as slow, rhythmic rotation and weight bearing, are useful. Air splints are often used to help with positioning, reduction of tone sensory awareness, or early gait training.

Discuss physical therapy interventions in the patient with a CVA related to performance of functional activities.

INTERVENTIONS FOR FUNCTIONAL ACTIVITIES

Functional movements should be taught as early as possible to a patient post-CVA. One of the first functional activities is rolling, both to the involved and uninvolved sides. Since the roll is initiated from the opposite side, rolling to the involved side is actually easier, but rolling to the uninvolved side can be aided by having the patient assume the hook lying position and grasping the hands together before rolling. The patient should learn to scoot in the supine position. Transfers should be taught, particularly supine-to-sit and wheelchair-to-bed/mat transfers. Supine-to-sit transfers should be learned on both the uninvolved and involved sides. Techniques include rolling onto the uninvolved side, followed by moving lower extremities off the bed; and a diagonal pattern, where the individual scoots to the edge through bridging, brings the lower extremities off the surface, and, while tucking the chin, reaches forward with the unaffected arm. The main wheelchair-to-bed/mat technique used is the stand-pivot transfer.

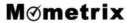

INTERVENTIONS FOR FUNCTIONAL POSITIONING

Once the patient post-CVA can accomplish short-sitting, which is sitting on the side of the bed or other surface with flexed knees and hips and feet planted on the floor, functional positioning can be addressed. The first interventions should concentrate on the patient's sitting posture, starting with guiding the pelvis through an anterior pelvic tilt, eventually into neutral, followed by positioning the trunk such that the shoulders are aligned over the hips, and positioning of the head upright. Adjunct sitting interventions include weight bearing on the involved hand, weight-shifting with arms resting in lap or bearing weight, sitting balance or isometric activities, reaching activities, and bilateral proprioceptive neuromuscular facilitation patterns performed seated. When possible, sit-to-stand transitions should be taught; these include techniques like standing in front of the patient with hands on the paraspinals to help them shift forward from sitting, guarding the patient from the involved side as they get up, and use of the uninvolved arm for independent transfers. Early standing activities should include weight-shifting with assistance in all four directions, while observing for posture, joint control, and balance.

AMBULATION PROGRESSION AND COMMON GAIT DEVIATIONS POST-CVA

The clinician helps the patient post-cerebrovascular accident through various stages to achieve ambulation. The initial stage, once the patient can stand, is to practice weight shifting in all four directions. The second is to have them learn to advance the uninvolved lower extremity both forward and backward with weight bearing, while blocking the involved leg to prevent knee buckling. After that the patient should be taught how to advance the involved leg forward; this may require tactile cues at the hip or the foot behind the patient by the PT or PTA. Extremity advancement steps are sometimes done with the patient seated. The next progression is stepping backward with the affected lower extremity, and the last step is putting several steps together, engaging both extremities. Advancing the involved leg during the swing phase and weight shifts during the stance phase of gait should be stressed. The patient normally uses a cane on the involved side, while the clinician provides support on the unaffected side, though recent studies are examining the long-term impact of cane use on the individual's gait symmetry. Common gait deviations to look for include hip retraction, hiking, circumduction, or inadequate flexion; knee instability, hyperextension, or undue flexion during stance or too little flexion during swing; and ankle inversion, eversion, footdrop, or toe clawing.

ADVANCED PHYSICAL THERAPY INTERVENTIONS

A natural progression in physical therapy interventions for patients experiencing a cerebrovascular accident or stroke is performance of prone activities; transitioning from prone on the elbows into the four-point or quadruped position; four-point activities, such as creeping; changing from the four-point into the tall-kneeling position; tall-kneeling activities, such as lifting; moving from tall-kneeling to half-kneeling; half-kneeling activities; and finally, the modified plant grade position. The latter is a standing position with weight bearing on all four extremities (for example, arms on a table); from this position, many types of exercises can be done, such as alternating isometrics, squats, or functional activities. During mid- to late recovery, physical therapy approaches include negotiation of stairs, both climbing and descending, with clinician assistance and wearing a safety belt; exercises to develop fine motor skills, coordination, and balance; and advanced exercises for ambulation-involved joints, especially the ankle. Useful equipment for balance exercises includes tilt boards and the Swiss ball.

PHYSICAL THERAPY FOR PATIENTS POST-TRAUMATIC BRAIN INJURY

In the acute period after medical stabilization, one of the most important considerations for patients with traumatic brain injuries (TBIs) is positioning. The best positioning for the patient post-TBI is not supine, but rather side-lying, semi-prone, or even prone, to reduce tonic labyrinthine reflexes. The prone position with various props is preferred for this patient using mechanical ventilation or a tracheostomy tube. Sensory stimulation and activities to increase patient awareness are indicated early. After the patient is transferred to an inpatient rehabilitation setting, the previously mentioned positioning should be continued along with some time spent in a wheelchair (regular or tilt-in-space type). Range-of-motion exercises should be begun, particularly stretching, as well as functional mobility training as patients typically lack postural and motor control post-TBI. Assisted sitting and standing activities and transfers should be incorporated. Activities addressing some of the associated cognitive deficits should be included when possible. Eventually, interventions can incorporate a variety of balance exercises using moving surfaces.

OUTPATIENT PHYSICAL THERAPY INTERVENTIONS

The goals of outpatient rehabilitation for patients with traumatic brain injuries center around improving outcomes related to physical impairments, activity limitations, and participation restrictions. Physical therapists develop treatment plans to help patients manage pain and impairments that may include cardiovascular function, strength, joint range of motion, muscle flexibility, spasticity, coordination, and balance. These plans are largely influenced by the severity of the injury and the patient's level of consciousness. Progressing with performance of functional transfers is a primary goal with the inclusion of patient education and training in the use of appropriate durable medical equipment. Where applicable, gait training is a key component of care to allow for access to areas inside and outside of the home. With an improvement in relevant impairments and activity limitations, physical therapists and their assistants are able to facilitate strategies for patient involvement in social activities with family and friends to work toward developing a higher quality of life.

PHYSICAL THERAPY FOR PATIENTS WITH SPINAL CORD INJURIES

ACUTE CARE PHYSICAL THERAPY

A good deal of physical therapy for patients with a spinal cord injury (SCI) in the acute setting should focus on improvement of respiratory function. This includes breathing exercises and diaphragmatic breathing in patients with C4 to T1 injuries, glossopharyngeal breathing for those with C1 to C3 damage, lateral expansion or basilar breathing in those with T1 to T12 injuries, incentive spirometry, manual chest stretching, postural drainage techniques, and assisted cough techniques. Acute care management should also focus on prevention of joint contractures, improvement of muscle function, prevention of other complications, and acclimation of the patient to the upright position (usually with a tilt table). Range-of-motion (ROM) exercises are essential, concentrating on stretching in upper regions and passive ROM in the lower paralyzed extremities. Strengthening exercises, usually employing manual resistance, should be performed.

INPATIENT REHABILITATION PHASE

Some of the earliest interventions for patients with a spinal cord injury during inpatient rehabilitation should be mat activities. Mat activities include the following:

- **Learning how to roll**: Flex and rotate head, extend arms above head, turn with momentum.
- **Exercises in prone position**: Scapular strengthening, for example.
- Transitions to prone on elbows.
- **Exercises in prone on elbows position**: For example, alternating isometrics.
- **Shifts from elbow position to supine**.
- **Transitions to supine on elbows**: Assisted or independent, utilizing neck shift forward and side weight shift to come onto the other elbow.
- **Movement from supine on elbows into long-sitting**: Extension of both lower extremities.

Another emphasis should be on how to perform transfers. Eventually patients with C7 tetraplegia should be taught how to self-stretch their hamstrings (in long-sitting or supine position), gluteus maximus, hip rotators, and ankle plantar flexors. Patients with paraplegia can move on to advanced mat activities, such as the sitting swing-through, hip swayer, trunk twisting and raising, prone push-ups, creeping, and tall-kneeling exercises with or without crutches. Other potential components include cardiopulmonary training, wheelchair use, circuit training, aquatic therapy, and for some, eventually, ambulation training.

OUTPATIENT PHYSICAL THERAPY INTERVENTIONS

The goals of outpatient rehabilitation for patients with spinal cord injuries center around improving physical impairments, improving tolerance and performance of activities of daily living, and the ability to participate meaningfully in social settings. Physical therapists develop treatment plans to help patients manage symptoms and improve their ability to function by developing their cardiovascular function, strength, range of motion, muscle flexibility, spasticity, coordination, and balance. Enhancing the patient's functional transfers to facilitate safe mobility through their environment is a primary goal with the inclusion of patient education and training in the use of appropriate durable medical equipment. Gait training is employed when appropriate to make sure patients are able to safely ambulate indoors and outdoors. Cognitive behavioral therapy is a psychotherapeutic approach that has been used to assist with treatment for chronic neuropathic pain as well as the psychosocial aspects of recovery from spinal cord injury. Physical therapists and their assistants are integral in facilitating the return of patient involvement in social activities, and in turn, allowing for a higher quality of life post-spinal cord injury.

PHYSICAL THERAPY INTERVENTIONS FOR PATIENTS WITH MULTIPLE SCLEROSIS

Most physical therapy interventions for patients with multiple sclerosis (MS) speak to the three major neurologic symptoms of weakness, spasticity, and ataxia.

- Exercises to address **weakness** should be performed at submaximal levels with interspersed rest periods to avoid fatigue. Strengthening is an important component, and should focus on high reps of low to moderate intensity. Low-level aerobics should be included. Patients should do exercises in a cool environment.
- In order to decrease the possibility of **spasticity** during exercise, slow static stretching exercises should be performed first. Examples include stretching of the heel cord and hamstrings, using a towel or assisted by the therapist; sitting and wall stretches for the hamstrings; stretching the legs against a wall to stretch hamstrings and hip adductors; rotating the lower trunk, using a therapy ball; and transiting from four-point to side sitting for trunk rotation.
- Interventions for **ataxia** should focus on postural exercises, functional movement transitions, static and dynamic balance training, and Frenkel exercises for coordination. Assistive devices or orthoses are often used.

PHYSICAL THERAPY INTERVENTIONS FOR PATIENTS WITH PARKINSON'S DISEASE

Early physical therapy interventions in patients with Parkinson's disease (PD) are imperative to maximize function. The approach is somewhat dependent on the predominant manifestation exhibited: bradykinesia, tremor, rigidity, postural instability, or the combined gait difficulty. Possible gait interventions include use of aids or cues to enhance attention; breaking down tasks into parts; working toward measurable goals, such as increasing stride length; and practicing different walking patterns. Some patients may need to use a walker or cane. Postural interventions include strengthening exercises for postural extensors, stretching of pectorals and heel cords, rotational exercises to increase range of motion of the neck and trunk (done while supine or side-

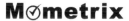

lying), and relaxation exercises, including deep breathing. Aerobic conditioning is also suggested to combat fatigue.

PHYSICAL THERAPY INTERVENTIONS FOR CHILDREN WITH CEREBRAL PALSY

The physical therapy examination for a child with cerebral palsy (CP) identifies their impairments and functional limitations within the context of the specific type of cerebral palsy in order to institute appropriate physical therapy. With the most common type, spastic cerebral palsy, typical impairments are increased muscle stiffness; slow movement, impacting balance and posture; decreased trunk rotation, making movement transitions difficult; decreased range of motion, affecting reaching and ambulation; skeletal malalignment and deformities; muscle weakness; and erroneous muscle recruitment. Physical therapy should focus on increased movement, righting and equilibrium exercises, protective reactions, movement transitions, skeletal positioning, use of orthoses, and muscle sequencing exercises. Patients with CP with athetosis or ataxia have postural instability due to low or fluctuating muscle tone, as well as uncoordinated movements; lack of midrange control, impacting reaching and walking; difficulty using their hands for support during transitions; a lack of graded movement, making it difficult to grasp or change positions; and emotional lability. Treatment should focus on holding postures, control of movements, holding midrange movements, upper-extremity weight bearing, stabilization, and behavior modification.